Rising Above Chronic Pain and Illness

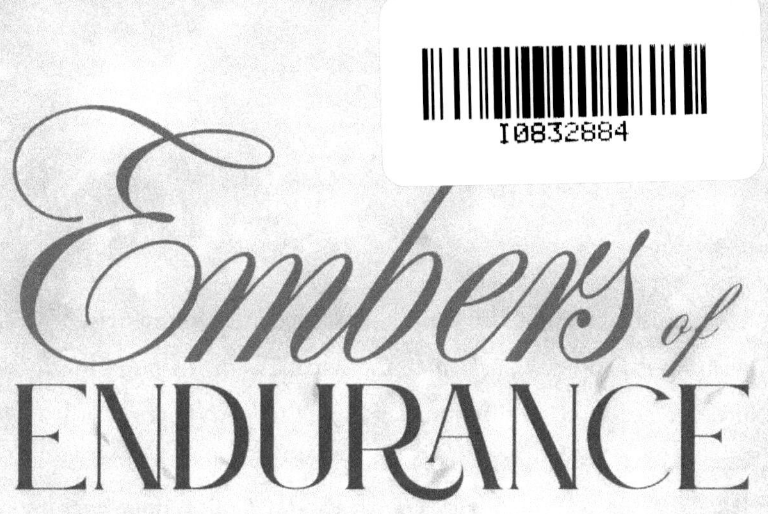

CAROLYN DALE NEWELL

What Others Are Saying

I just finished reading this book and immediately found myself wishing it had been handed to me when I went through my massive health crisis this summer. I will refer to it often as I struggle to run the race of chronic health issues with endurance. Page after page is filled with raw truth and biblical hope that encourages and heals. Carolyn writes from the perspective of one who's been on the ash pile and has risen above the embers to spiritual victory. Highly recommend to all who sit on the ash pile.

Dr. Mel Tavares, editor of *Arise Daily*,
an EPA award-winning digital devotional platform

What I appreciate about *Embers of Endurance* is its honesty. Carolyn Dale Newell doesn't offer easy answers or quick spiritual fixes. Instead, she offers Scripture, compassion, and the reassurance that God is still present when healing is slow—or doesn't come the way we hoped.

This book is a steady companion for anyone living with chronic pain or illness, reminding us that God has not abandoned us and that endurance itself can become a place of grace.

Linda Evans Shepherd, founder of Advanced Writers & Speakers Association and author of *Praying the Word: 90 Scripture-Powered Prayers to Calm an Anxious Heart*

Embers of Endurance meets readers in the sacred space between pain and uncertainty, all the while offering the steady assurance that God never leaves us alone in our hurt. With humility and unflinching honesty, Carolyn Dale Newell does not discount the hard of chronic, physical suffering but tenderly guides our hearts back to His truth, His hope, and His grace. A gentle companion for weary souls, this book beckons us to believe that beauty can still rise from ashes, even when the road is long and dark.

Sara Cormany, award-winning author of *Even When: Experiencing God's Presence on Difficult Days*

This thirty-day devotional is a lifeline for anyone walking through a difficult season. Even when your faith feels unsteady, these pages gently guide you back to the unshakable truth of God's Word. Each devotion is filled with encouragement, strength, and the reminder that victory is still possible, no matter what you're facing. This book doesn't just inspire faith; it rebuilds it, day by day. A must-read for anyone seeking hope, clarity, and renewed confidence in God's promises.

Evelyn Johnson-Taylor, Ph.D, professor, author, and speaker

Carolyn Dale Newell's vulnerability about her own journey through relentless pain gives us permission to struggle while still believing, to question while still trusting. If you're exhausted by well-meaning advice that doesn't match your reality, read this book. *Embers of Endurance* is a beautifully written lifeline for anyone who's tired of spiritual platitudes and desperately needs someone who understands that faith and suffering can—and often *must*—coexist.

Carol Kent, speaker and author of *When I Lay My Isaac Down* (NavPress) and *He Holds My Hand* (Tyndale)

More Books by Carolyn

Incense Rising: 60 Days to Powerful Prayer

Overcoming the Overwhelming:
Walking in Victorious Faith When You Don't Feel Victorious

Eyes of Faith:
Winning the Battle Between Your Feelings and Your Faith

Faith, Freedom and 4 Paws:
Seeing God Through Iva's Eyes (Guide Dog Tales Book One)

Walking By Faith Not Sight:
30 Inspirational Moments with Iva
(Guide Dog Tales Book Two)

Faith That Walks on Water:
Conquering Emotional Bondage with the Armor of God

EMBERS OF ENDURANCE

Rising Above Chronic Pain and Illness

Interior & Cover Design by Ruth Hovsepian

BEATITUDES PUBLISHING

Paperback ISBN: 978-1-962581-84-4

eBook ISBN: 978-1-962581-85-1

I dedicate this book to my aunt, Dorothy Anderson Camden, and my cousin, Pamela Anderson. I miss you both dearly, but I will see you again in Heaven.

To console those who mourn in Zion,

To give them beauty for ashes,

The oil of joy for mourning,

The garment of praise for the spirit of heaviness;

That they may be called trees of righteousness,

The planting of the Lord, that He may be glorified.

Isaiah 61:3 NKJV

Contents

Introduction

As we struggle with chronic pain or illness, another struggle lies deep inside. It affects us emotionally, mentally, and spiritually, and it stems from discouragement. We become discouraged when our prayers go unanswered, the doctors can't give us a diagnosis, or the next appointment isn't soon enough.

While discouragement had its tentacles wrapped tightly around me, it seemed easier for doubt to chisel away at my faith. Before I realized it, I was depressed, living without joy and peace. Life seemed hopeless because surgery changed my life forever.

Once God brought me out of the darkness, I found Scriptures I'd never given much attention. Job and the psalmist felt like I did. Elijah gave up and couldn't resist the threat to his life. I was in good company, and so are you, my friend.

It's all right if your faith feels shaky today. I have found biblical and practical ways to stabilize our faith. I realized that I walked a horrific journey of pain due to scoliosis in order to share my experience with you.

These devotions aren't filled with one victory after another but rather a slow, steady pace to living like the conquerors God has made each of us to be.

I felt like my life was a pile of ashes, but then embers began to rise above that pile. Something sparked in my life. God gives us beauty for ashes, and I want to help you find beautiful again.

I'm glad you are reading this book, because I have prayed for you as I pounded words out on my laptop. I will continue to pray as these words leave my computer and become the book you hold in your hands. It will not only encourage you but transform your outlook and mindset as you traverse your own health problems.

While reading, you will gain hope, rest in joy and peace, and discover how to walk with spiritual endurance. Once you finish, you will know the Scriptures to keep close to your heart and recognize the hand of the enemy as he tries to pull you back into despair.

You will no longer give in to what you go through. You will realize God hasn't stopped working or forgotten you, but He is sovereignly working in the dark.

This book cannot change your pain or illness, but it will change your spirit and soul as you navigate your own traumatic health crisis.

Are you ready to get started? Just turn the page and start a new page of your life.

Rising Above Chronic Pain and Illness

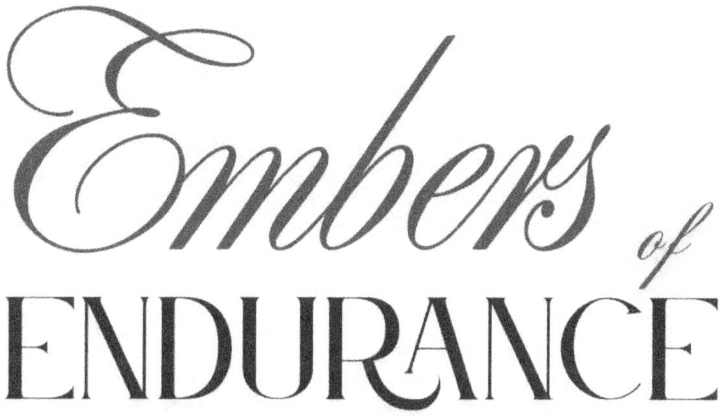

CAROLYN DALE NEWELL

Day 1

Don't Lose Your Fight

No weapon formed against you shall prosper,
And every tongue which rises against you in judgment
You shall condemn.
Isaiah 54:17 NKJV

"No weapon formed against me shall prosper!" I declared this verse with determination while watering my bright yellow mums. As I gave each vibrant plant a cool drink, my back pain intensified. Spiritual warfare comes with publishing another book, but I was ready to fight. One more flower, and I could go inside and rest on my heating pad.

I'm no stranger to back pain, but suddenly I felt something unusual. A sharp pain shot from my back, into my hip, and down my leg. I dropped to my knees, and the tears began.

Each morning and evening, I had met with the Lord in prayer. My faith was on fire, and I had plenty of fight in me. Over the next two years, chronic pain and illness diminished that flame, and the fight disappeared.

Excruciating pain, great disappointment, and depression beat me down. I still uttered a prayer for relief, but they were merely words with little passion.

God is sovereign in our pain. This means He always has total control of our lives. We see the clearest picture of His sovereignty in the first two chapters of Job.

It might seem like God threw Job under the bus when God asked Satan if he had considered Job, a blameless man (Job 1:8). Satan told God that Job was only righteous because God hedged him all around (Job 1:10). Satan suggested that if God touched all Job had, he would curse God (Job 1:11).

"And the Lord said to Satan, 'Behold, all that he has is in your power; only do not lay a hand on his person.' So Satan went out from the presence of the Lord" (Job 1:12 NKJV).

God, in His sovereignty, allows suffering. He allowed Job to lose his children, servants, and flocks. Sometimes, He allows the devil to sift us like wheat, but God also allows trials in our lives for our growth. God wants us to be like Christ. It's the devil's dirty plan, but God allows it and makes beneficial use of it, even though it may be painful for us.

Suffering doesn't always come at the hands of the enemy. Suffering increases our faith, but pain tempts us to lose our fight, the willpower to resist the enemy. Whether we fight the enemy in prayer, or we fight for healing, something deep inside pushes us to find this illness unacceptable.

Let's keep our doctrine straight when it comes to what the enemy does. The devil isn't winning, and God hasn't stopped helping us.

God isn't surprised at the horrible things happening in your life. He hears your cries. While God is silent, He is still there. He is still in control. The victory was won over two thousand years ago on the cross.

I don't know where your journey has taken you, but I want to sit next to you and take your hand. Blindness prevents me from looking you straight in the eye as I tell you, "Don't lose your fight."

Your journey already feels treacherous, or perhaps it has just begun, but hang on to hope. Keep your eyes on Jesus, and if the waves pull you under, get Him back in your focus as soon as you catch your next breath.

Our verse from Isaiah is true. The weapon of crippling pain was formed, but it did not prosper. I am walking again without much pain, but the weapon was formed, and it did beat me down. Yet, it never prospered. Devil, do you hear that? It never prospered.

It might get rough for you, but that weapon won't prosper. We fight *from* victory, not *for* victory. Jesus has already won your battle. You are guaranteed eternal life with Jesus if you are a believer. Don't lose your fight.

Reading and praying through the Psalms greatly helped me. They offer amazing comfort, and they show us we're not alone. Many nights, I read one after another until I fell asleep. I know they will encourage you.

I rise before the dawning of the morning,
And cry for help;
I hope in Your word.
Psalm 119:147 NKJV

Lord, You are my healer. I believe You can heal me this moment, and I also understand You are sovereign. May Your will be done, in the name of Jesus Christ. Amen.

Day 2

When Helplessness Intrudes

Fear not, for I am with you;
Be not dismayed, for I am your God.
I will strengthen you,
Yes, I will help you,
I will uphold you with My righteous right hand.
Isaiah 41:10 NKJV

I learned these sharp pains shooting from my back down my leg are called sciatica, according to the internet. I was self-diagnosing.

I thought, "I must continue moving forward with all the things necessary to publish a book. God must intervene because this pain could last for several weeks. I don't have time for that! I have a book signing scheduled for our local fall festival in a few weeks. I also have a speaking event approaching."

The heating pad barely comforted the incredible pain, and fear began to set off all kinds of alarms.

I went to my primary care doctor. As he sent prescriptions to the pharmacy on his computer, he explained, "Sciatica is a symptom of something else, so we must find out what that is. I'm ordering X-rays."

I had the X-rays, and I couldn't believe what the nurse said when she called. "You have spinal stenosis, and there is no surgery for it. The doctor wants you to get an MRI and go to physical therapy."

I went back to the internet searching for a treatment, but I found nothing. Both my pain and feelings of helplessness increased. Was physical therapy my only available treatment? Why hadn't God intervened?

God is our strength and help in times of fear and confusion. We have no reason to be afraid of the unknown or a bad diagnosis because God is with us. He never leaves us. No matter how gruesome the pain becomes or how our world changes, we can count on God.

Look at today's verse. God tells us not to fear. This is intricately woven throughout Scripture. God knows how hard it is for us to avoid fear. It paralyzes us, and when we are fearful, it's difficult to have faith. Next, God says we shouldn't be dismayed. This has the connotation of discouragement or disheartenment. We deal with all these feelings throughout life, especially during illness.

Then God reminds us He is our God. He is supreme and sovereign. He is our loving Father who strengthens us. We can take our fear, discouragement, and weakness to God and rely on His strength when we lack our own.

God says He will help us. We have the supreme ruler of the universe as our helper. We also have the Holy Spirit indwelling us. We are blessed beyond measure, and He upholds us with His right hand, which refers to power.

This might be a good verse to memorize because it is filled with the power of God.

How can you press into God as you meditate on this verse?

Psalm 10:14 (NKJV) says, "The helpless commits himself to you [God]."

Fear and confusion are normal when medical professionals cannot give us a plan of action, but we can't allow these feelings to consume us. Our flesh tends to feed on fear, and the enemy uses this for his own purposes.

In anxious times, we must commit to trust God. When doctors can't help, God can. When the diagnosis sounds horrible, God has a plan. When doors don't open, God holds the key.

What's creating fear in your life? What doesn't make sense and frustrates you? Our flesh wants to sulk in these emotions, but we must remove ourselves from these feelings. They cannot dictate our lives.

Take extra time in prayer and the Word of God. This is where you meet with your Helper, and He renews your strength. He will build up your faith and cast away your fears.

What has God done for you in the past? Count those blessings. He healed my husband from leukemia. He carried me through depression. He healed my hearing loss when doctors did all they could do. He can come through for you now, my friend.

Bless the Lord, O my soul,
And forget not all His benefits:
Who forgives all your iniquities,
Who heals all your diseases,
Who redeems your life from destruction.
Psalm 103:2–4 NKJV

Heavenly Father, I am afraid and helpless, but You are my divine help. I believe You will remove my fears and give me wisdom. Help me hold onto You in these difficult days. In Jesus's name. Amen.

Day 3

A Shot of Joy

Then he said to them, "Go your way, eat the fat,
drink the sweet, and send portions to those for
whom nothing is prepared; for this day is holy to our Lord.
Do not sorrow, for the joy of the Lord is your strength."
Nehemiah 8:10 NKJV

Wouldn't it be wonderful if we could receive a shot of joy? Before I left his office, the doctor gave me two injections for pain, and it might as well have been a shot of joy.

The injections worked quickly, spreading much welcome relief throughout my body. As soon as I returned home, I wanted to go for a walk with my guide dog, a beautiful black Labrador retriever named Iva. I put the harness on her with much excitement. Iva and I hadn't walked for several days because of my intense pain.

As we walked on that beautiful fall afternoon, I noticed that Iva sensed my joy. I was thrilled to walk without pain when, just that morning, I couldn't do it. Iva had missed our walks as much as I had. When we returned to the house, I felt drowsy from the injections, but I wasn't ready to end our walk. We continued our walk on the street in front of our house until I had to go inside and sleep it off.

When I woke up, I remembered the pain had disappeared, but when I moved, a sharp pain quickly reminded me it had returned. That was the last day I walked Iva for three months.

The Holy Spirit infuses us with joy because joy strengthens us. Today's verse comes from the book of Nehemiah, where we find weeping and sorrow. The Hebrews gathered to hear the reading of God's Word, and it sliced their hearts. Their eyes were opened to their sin and rebellion, and they were overwhelmed with grief.

They repented, and God didn't want them to continue mourning for their actions. Instead, He wanted them to celebrate that day, give gifts, and choose joy. They needed strength to rebuild Jerusalem, and the joy of the Lord gives us strength.

They found joy in the Word of God when they understood it. They found joy in repentance.

The devil wants to steal our joy. He can't steal our salvation, but he can make us miserable Christians, and that's not a good testimony to the world.

We find joy in God's Word and in prayer. God also gives us simple things to remind us of His joy. It may be a gentle breeze while you sit outside, a comfy recliner to rest in, an afternoon nap, family and friends, or a walk with your dog. Psalm 30:5 (NKJV) says, "Weeping may endure for a night, but joy *comes* in the morning."

Did you know it is normal to mourn the loss of our health? I didn't lose most of my vision until age fifty, and then it declined rapidly. Counselors told me it was normal to grieve that loss. It was normal to grieve my inability to walk. It's normal for you to grieve the lack you are experiencing today.

Like grief over a loved one who passes, we weep for a season, but then joy returns. Don't get caught up in the grief. Choose joy!

Strength flows from the springs of joy. The joy of the Lord gives us strength. That's why the enemy strives to destroy it.

What gives you joy? I had to start walking with a cane shortly after that day, but I longed to walk with Iva again. It became my goal in healing. It gave me the strength to keep going.

Do you have a goal you are working toward? How do you find strength from joy?

I am closing with Isaiah 35:10. Can we be like these Israelites and rejoice always? Sorrows will flee. My friend, I have lost joy at times, and it's easier to never let it slip out of our hands. Rekindle the fire of joy in your life today.

And those the Lord has rescued will return.
They will enter Zion with singing;
everlasting joy will crown their heads.
Gladness and joy will overtake them,
and sorrow and sighing will flee away.
Isaiah 35:10 (NIV)

Heavenly Father, help me choose joy in the little things, even though I am sick and in pain. Help me work toward attainable goals and infuse me with joy, which is my strength. In Jesus's name. Amen.

Day 4

God Never Promised Easy

I can do all things through Christ who strengthens me.
Philippians 4:13 NKJV

I agonized as I willed my body out of bed. With my feet firmly planted on the floor, I had to take a step. Do you remember the tin man in the movie, *The Wizard of Oz*? He rusted and couldn't move until Dorothy or the Scarecrow oiled him up. I felt like I needed his oil can.

After making it to the bathroom, it would be easier to return to bed, but I knew I had to walk off the stiffness. I hobbled down the hallway hunched over my cane.

Some mornings, I could barely take a step. My husband stood in front of me, and I held onto his shoulders. He took slow, definite steps, and we walked up and down the hallway until some of the stiffness wore off. Then I returned to bed with an ice pack, and my husband rubbed my back and hip with a topical pain reliever.

From my bed, I completed a speaking certificate via Zoom, and I launched my book, *Faith That Walks on Water*.

I went to physical therapy several times a week. Getting in and out of the car sent shocks of pain through my body. Just sitting in the car was miserable. How would I ever make the forty-minute trip to the imaging center for the MRI?

I finally decided to travel by lying down in the back seat. That worked, but once I made it to the MRI table, severe pain prevented me from pulling my other leg onto the table. The nurses tried to lift my leg, but with each attempt, my screams frightened them.

I couldn't see a spine surgeon without an MRI, so I had to get through it. The results didn't offer any conclusive answers, but at least I could see a surgeon and find out if they could help me. By this point, I didn't want to avoid surgery. I couldn't live in this pain, barely able to walk.

God strengthens us, but He never promised to make it easy. We don't know what we will have to endure. Can you imagine going through difficulties without His strength?

For some reason, we think His strength will make life easy. That's not true. Just above this verse, the apostle Paul spoke about learning to be content in any situation. He wrote about hunger and suffering. Paul's life wasn't easy, but he made it through all the trials with strength from Jesus Christ.

That same strength is available to us. Jesus said, "These things I have spoken to you, that in Me you may have peace. In the world you will have tribulation; but be of good cheer, I have overcome the world" (John 16:33 NKJV).

In this verse, Jesus promised tribulations while we live in this world. Tribulations aren't easy. He also promised peace and encouraged us to be of good cheer. *The Christian Standard Bible (CSB)* translates this as "be courageous."

With His strength, I tried being courageous.

I don't know the severity of your pain or illness, but I know it isn't easy. As you go through your day, declare these Scriptures. They will encourage you and help you believe you are walking in the strength of Christ, difficult as it may be.

Don't allow fear to taunt you. Jesus has overcome fear. He has overcome the devil. He has overcome death, and He has overcome this world. Take courage in that. He has already won the victory. You're just waiting for the outcome.

Seek peace during your day. Which things chase away the anxiety? Perhaps worship music, a bubble bath, or sitting outside listening to the birds sing. Be kind to yourself, keep praying, and refresh your peace. Prayer is the lifeline to God's power.

I challenge you to do one thing each day to treat yourself and soak in the peace of Jesus. This journey is hard, but with Christ, you can make it.

Not that I speak in regard to need, for I have
learned in whatever state I am, to be content.
Philippians 4:11 NKJV

Heavenly Father, You promised me strength and peace, but they escape me in the mess I'm in. Please give me a break where I can feel Your presence, and let peace rule over my heart and mind. Give me the strength for the next thing. In Jesus's name. Amen.

Day 5

Another Cancellation

Yet the chief butler did not remember Joseph, but forgot him.
Genesis 40:23 NKJV

"Hi, I'm sorry, but I am not able to speak at your event." I had to make that same phone call several times during the fall of 2022, due to relentless pain. Sadly, I had to cancel events again in August 2024, after a gall bladder surgery.

Everyone understood. Everyone but me, that is. I don't like change, and I hate interruptions. That's all my life had become—one big interruption.

I hated the devil, and I couldn't understand how this could be part of God's plan. Perhaps you have felt like that when your life has been put on hold.

Why couldn't the doctors treat this horrific pain? Why wasn't it getting better with physical therapy? Why didn't God heal me? Instead, I limped around, screaming in pain whenever I tried to get in a car or lie down.

I reminded myself God had better plans. I didn't want to fall deep into the darkness of depression. I also didn't want to be angry with God. I needed Him, so I refused to be angry at anyone but myself and the doctors.

Just when my ministry was taking off after the pandemic, my world fell apart. Not just part of my world, but all of it. Wasn't it enough that I was blind? I could live with blindness but not with this pain.

Joseph's life was interrupted for thirteen years. It began when his jealous brothers sold him to slave traders traveling to Egypt. Once in Egypt, he obtained a good job with Potiphar, who threw Joseph into prison when his wife made false allegations about Joseph taking liberties with her.

In prison, Joseph had favor with the prison guard, and he met two of Pharaoh's staff: the butler and baker. They each had dreams that disturbed them. Joseph was an interpreter of dreams and volunteered to help them.

Sadly, the baker was executed, but the butler was released. Joseph begged him to remember him because he didn't belong in prison. The butler promised Joseph he would speak favorably about him and help him with his release, but he forgot about Joseph.

Once again, Joseph's life continued on a detour until Pharaoh had some disturbing dreams that none of his magicians could interpret.

The butler recalled Joseph, and he told Pharaoh about Joseph's skills. Pharaoh sent for Joseph, and he moved up from the prison to the palace. He soon became second in command over Egypt.

Do you think Joseph was confused by the interruptions in his life? It doesn't seem like part of God's plan. Why would God allow such a long separation from his beloved father? You've thought the same thing, wondering when life will return to normal.

Defeat overwhelms us when our bodies force us to cancel plans. We feel like our bodies have failed us, although it's truly bad timing. These bodies are just dust. Perhaps you know the disappointment of an interrupted life. It changes your plans as discouragement takes over.

God is sovereign. He controls all things, and He has plans we cannot understand. If the enemy has laid a hand on us, it is only because God has allowed it in order for His purposes.

Daniel 4:35 (NIV) says, "All the peoples of the earth are regarded as nothing. He does as he pleases with the powers of heaven and the peoples of the earth. No one can hold back his hand or say to him: 'What have you done?'"

Our loving Father is good toward us. He also works things together for good. While all things are not good, God weaves them into the tapestry of our lives to use them for good.

Spend some time thanking God for His goodness today. Grasp onto God's sovereignty and trust Him while your life is being turned upside down. Do you think Joseph ever realized how his suffering could encourage so many of us? How can your trial be an encouragement for someone else?

The Lord bestows favor and honor;
no good thing does he withhold
from those whose walk is blameless.
Psalm 84:11 NIV

Heavenly Father, I don't understand the turn my life has taken, but I believe You are good and in control of all things, so I choose to trust You. In Jesus's name. Amen.

Day 6

Will God Give You Too Much to Handle?

No temptation has overtaken you except such as is common to man; but God *is* faithful, who will not allow you to be tempted beyond what you are able, but with the temptation will also make the way of escape, that you may be able to bear it.
1 Corinthians 10:13 NKJV

I felt the ultimate helplessness lying in bed with an ice pack, unable to assist my husband while he took care of me and his dying mother. Pain confined me to my bed and recliner for three months. On the Sunday before Thanksgiving, my husband, Timmy, went to check on his elderly mom, who lives next door. I wondered what kept him so long.

When he came home, my heart broke for him. He had found his mom lying on the floor, unable to get up. She refused to let him call the rescue squad or take her to the emergency room. Within a few days, he realized she was dying, and he didn't know how to help her. All week, he ran back and forth, taking care of his mother and me. Our church helped tremendously with meals that week.

Timmy insisted on having a small Thanksgiving dinner, even though our lives were chaotic. He fixed a turkey breast and some vegetables, and I hobbled to the kitchen to eat. It was quiet and nice.

Timmy's mom peacefully passed away in her sleep that weekend. My husband needed me, but how could I stand by his side while I was in so much pain? I went with him to make arrangements at the funeral home. Like a jack-in-the-box, I sprang up and down on the chair. Neither sitting nor standing gave me any relief from the nerve shocks traveling from my back to my leg.

At the funeral, people helped me from the car to my seat. How would I sit on that folding aluminum chair during the entire service? The pastor leaned over and assured me in a gentle voice he would keep it short. God miraculously allowed me to sit for the entire service without pain.

God gives us more than we can bear because He helps us bear it. Otherwise, we would never need Him. Many people, including myself, make our focal verse sound like God never gives us more than we can handle. If that were the case, we wouldn't cry out to Him for help so often. When we look at this verse with that perspective, we are taking the verse out of context.

In the Bible, the Greek word "*peirasmos*" is either translated as trial or temptation. What makes a trial a temptation is the way we handle it. We begin doubting God. We may even fall into sin because we cannot handle the pressure of the trial.

If you turn to 1 Corinthians 10 and read the entire chapter, you will realize the apostle Paul is speaking about sin when he uses the word temptation. In this chapter, Paul discusses the sins of the wilderness-wandering Israelites, such as lusting after evil things, idolatry, and sexual immorality (1 Corinthians 10:68).

Today's verse tells us we aren't ever tempted by something new. We face the same temptations as other people. God will not allow us to be tempted beyond what we can bear. This refers to a temptation to sin, not enduring a trial. He will always make an escape for us to avoid sin.

Look in the middle of that verse. God is faithful! He is faithful when we are tempted to sin. He is also faithful during our most difficult trials. When we are weak, He makes us strong (2 Corinthians 12:10).

What are you going through today? Is it more than you can handle? Sweet friend, with God, you can handle it. It's never easy, but God is faithful.

When I came to the point where I lost all hope, God remained faithful. When joy and peace disappeared, God stayed faithful. When my faith wavered, God was faithful.

Meditate on the faithfulness of God today. What has He brought you through? Begin by giving Him thanks.

Beloved, do not think it strange concerning the
fiery trial which is to try you, as though some
strange thing happened to you.
1 Peter 4:12 NKJV

Heavenly Father, this is more than I can bear, but You are faithful. You strengthen me. You cover me with Your grace like a blanket. In Jesus's name. Amen.

Day 7

Next Steps

But those who wait on the Lord
Shall renew *their* strength;
They shall mount up with wings like eagles,
They shall run and not be weary,
They shall walk and not faint.
Isaiah 40:31 NKJV

"This doctor does surgery on spinal stenosis. He did it for me," my friend encouraged me. It was hard to understand how one doctor does the surgery when my primary care doctor and most of the internet say no surgery exists for that condition.

I had to jump through hoops to get the appointment with the spine surgeon: X-rays, physical therapy, and an MRI. Nothing had helped. The only place I found relief was in bed with an ice pack.

Once I made the appointment, it seemed like an eternity away. The spine center was about an hour away, so I lay down in the back seat of our car for the long trip, since sitting remained unbearable. I impatiently waited for the nurse to call my name while I bounced from my seat to standing to pacing back and forth in the waiting room. By this time, every position grew more painful.

The doctor sounded optimistic, but insurance required me to jump through more hoops. First, I had to endure two epidurals, and I begged them to give me the first one that day, but they didn't have any openings. Thankfully, they scheduled both epidurals before Christmas. I hoped they would offer all the relief I needed, and I could avoid surgery.

It had been almost three months since the day crippling pain attacked my body. I wanted relief. I wanted to walk again, especially with Iva. I wanted my life back. Can you relate?

God works while we wait. Waiting is part of God's plan, and I am not a fan of waiting, especially where pain is concerned. Since you are reading this book, you are probably in a season of waiting. How well do you handle waiting?

Perhaps waiting feels like wasted time. It appears as if nothing productive is happening, but God works in the background while we wait. He may be working on a doctor or the person you will witness to in the hospital. He also works on us. Not necessarily to bring healing, but He works on our character. He makes us more like Christ.

Isaiah penned today's verse while reminding Israel about the greatness of God during a time when they felt defeated. Defeat causes us to feel weary in our times of waiting. This verse tells us God renews our strength while we wait. According to Warren Wiersbe, the word renew means to exchange.[1] We need to exchange our feelings of defeat and weakness for God's strength.

I love this verse, and over the years, I have learned some magnificent facts about eagles. Their wing span averages about seven feet, and they have the strength to carry large bodies of prey. They can also fly at speeds of forty miles per hour.

With all their majesty and impressive strength, eagles rely on a force rather than their own strength. They lift their wings and allow air currents to carry them.

Friend, if a bird with the strength of an eagle relies on the wind, how much more do we need the Holy Spirit to carry us? God wants us to depend on Him while trusting Him in our seasons of waiting.

I could barely walk, so running without weariness seemed impossible, but I kept taking the next steps. I took the next step from the doctor to the epidural. Each morning, I took the next steps down the hallway, working out the stiffness. My pain was great, but God is greater.

---

1. Warren W. Wiersbe, *Be Comforted(Isaiah): Feeling Secure in the Arms of God (The BE Series Commentary)* (David C. Cook, 2009), Chapter 9. Kindle.

That's what Isaiah tells us in this verse. Wait on God. He will strengthen us. Depend on His strength. No matter how weak you feel, don't lose your hope. I know the waiting is hard, but God works while we wait.

I wait for the Lord, my soul waits,
And in His word I do hope.
My soul *waits* for the Lord
More than those who watch for the morning—
Yes, more than those who watch for the
morning.
Psalm 130:5–6 NKJV

Heavenly Father, I remind myself You are working while I am waiting. Strengthen me as I wait. Strengthen my hope, so I don't grow faint. In Jesus's name. Amen.

Day 8

When God's Grace Doesn't Feel Sufficient

Concerning this thing I pleaded with the Lord three times that it might depart from me. And He said to me, "My grace is sufficient for you, for My strength is made perfect in weakness." Therefore most gladly I will rather boast in my infirmities, that the power of Christ may rest upon me.
2 Corinthians 12:8–9 NKJV

"God, I don't mean to be disrespectful, but Your grace doesn't feel very sufficient right now. I'm thinking it, and You know my thoughts, so I might as well say it. Your grace isn't sufficient this time."

After that bold prayer, I continued whimpering in pain upon my bed. It had become my office. Whenever I sat anywhere, sharp pains nagged at me until I had to get up and return to my bed. I couldn't sit at my desk for Zoom meetings. Sitting at the kitchen table made eating unenjoyable with the recurring sharp pains. The sofa and recliner created the most pain, so my bed was my main location for several months.

Where was the all-sufficient grace God promised? Pain became my single focus. My eyes weren't on Jesus, or I would have witnessed His amazing grace in abundance. Focus on Christ, not the crisis.

Didn't God give me air to breathe and voice my complaints? Hadn't Jesus suffered and died so I could become a member of His family? How would I feel if my ice pack and medications were removed? What if I didn't have a home or bed to rest on while I whined?

Have you ever felt like God's grace wasn't enough? Have you ever wondered when that grace would kick in? Perhaps you showed more reverence than me, and you never voiced your thoughts, but it had crossed your mind.

God's supply of grace is unlimited. Paul had a major problem, which he referred to as a thorn in the flesh. Paul was given a thorn to keep him humble (2 Corinthians 12:7). He asked God to remove it three times. Paul didn't want to give up, but God refused. He told Paul, "My grace is sufficient for you, for My strength is made perfect in weakness" (2 Corinthians 12:9). God gave Paul the sufficient grace he needed to live with the thorn.

In Paul's weakness, God's strength was made perfect. Paul had to live with his thorn, but God gave him enough grace to deal with it.

Paul rejoiced over this grace. We see his joy in 2 Corinthians 12:10 (NKJV): "Therefore I take pleasure in infirmities, in reproaches, in needs, in persecutions, in distresses, for Christ's sake. For when I am weak, then I am strong."

I'm glad we don't know what Paul's thorn was because it could be the same thorn I have. It could be your thorn.

Several minutes passed, and I stopped begging God to help. In those moments of silence, a peace surrounded me. I even experienced some temporary relief from the pain. God's grace truly is sufficient. How could I have complained?

Perhaps He waits for us to ask for His help. Perhaps He waits for us to stop complaining. If we didn't have a thorn, we would never need His grace. We would never know what it is like to cry out for grace, God's unmerited favor.

What thorn do you have now? Have you seen God's grace? Are you like me, and you don't recognize His grace? Is your focus on your pain and illness rather than Christ? I certainly understand if it is. Pain and sickness are impossible to ignore. I feel sure you have already asked God to touch your body and remove your thorn. That's probably why you're reading this book. Now ask Him for His awesome grace.

If God hasn't removed your thorn, it doesn't mean He never will. I lived with various levels of pain for a long time. I still deal with some residual pain. Never stop praying for the healing touch of our Great Physician unless you know without a doubt that His answer is no. Like the psalmist, plead your case and watch expectantly for His answer.

In the morning, Lord, you hear my voice;
in the morning I plead my case to you
and watch expectantly.
Psalm 5:3 CSB

Lord God, You have promised sufficient grace for me in my seasons of thorns. Please let me see Your sufficient grace right now. Help me keep my eyes on You. I plead my case, and I watch for my healing. In Jesus's name. Amen.

Day 9

How Long?

Have mercy on me, O Lord, for I *am* weak;
O Lord, heal me, for my bones are troubled.
My soul also is greatly troubled;
But You, O Lord—how long?
Psalm 6:2–3 NKJV

I fought through constant pain, waiting for something to change. If the pain doesn't wear you down, the waiting will. I longed for normal again.

None of that mattered as much as being able to walk Iva again. I can't describe the relationship between a guide dog and handler, but as much as my body ached with pain, my heart ached for Iva. She stayed with me on my bed. When I screamed, she rushed to lick my face.

Would the epidural make a difference? I feared having a needle in my back, but I was desperate. I couldn't have surgery without first having the two epidurals.

Once again, I lay down in the back seat to travel the hour-long drive to the spine center. The needle didn't cause the pain, but when the medicine reached my inflamed leg, I screamed like crazy. It felt worse than my nerve shocks because it was unceasing.

"I can't take any more!"

They stopped short of injecting all the medicine, because I couldn't bear the pain. The doctor said, "Your pain tells us we hit the right spot."

"I'm sorry, but I couldn't handle it any longer."

I felt the difference in my pain level the next morning, as I could move easier. I could even sit some. I had one more injection just before Christmas, but it didn't help me enough to rule out surgery. The injections improved my mobility by about seventy-five percent, but I still needed surgery after the new year. Then this could all be over, or at least that's what I thought.

I delighted in my new mobility, and I attended church for the first time in three months. It was the Christmas service. Sitting and standing still created pain, but I made it through the entire service.

David suffered with pain as he cried out to God. He begged God not to rebuke him in His anger (Psalm 6:1). Perhaps his trial was some form of chastisement, but that's not always the reason for suffering.

While David suffered physically, his soul was troubled. Physical pain and illness affect every part of our lives, including our mental, emotional, and even our spiritual health.

I'm sure you have asked, "How long?" When pain drags on, we wonder if God will ever heal us. We wonder how long it will take Him to give us relief. It never crosses our minds to ask God what He wants us to gain from this trial, while we groan in agony, like David (Psalm 6:6).

David soaked his bed with tears. Does that sound familiar? We don't know how long it took God to heal David, but in verse nine, we read that the Lord has heard his prayer. It seems as if his troubles have been resolved.

We don't see David giving up, and neither can we. Many times, I felt praying was a useless repetition. I never turned away from God, but I grew weary in praying. After my surgery, life became so dark that I uttered words without much thought, but I never gave up, although I came really close.

God has a purpose for our suffering, and reasons for every sleepless night and every tear we cry. We cannot understand His ways, nor His timing. This is when trusting God gets hard, but don't give up.

God hears your prayers. He sees your tears. Jesus lived as a man on this earth, and He suffered more pain than we know when

He gave up His life for ours. Life is filled with pain, and the Christian life is no different.

Pain puts us in a situation where we cry out to God. It helps us become more like Christ. God works on us in our suffering.

Once the trial ends, our faith has been refined through the fire. Believe your Heavenly Father is listening to your cries. Don't give up. David wrote in verse 9 (NKJV), "The Lord has heard my supplication; The Lord will receive my prayer."

Heavenly Father, I cry out for healing once again. I agonize in my body and my soul. Thank You for hearing, and have mercy on me. In Jesus's name. Amen.

Day 10

Don't Let the Enemy Take Your Life

And a woman was there who had been
subject to bleeding for twelve years.
She had suffered a great deal under the
care of many doctors and had spent all she had,
yet instead of getting better she grew worse.
Mark 5:25–26 NIV

Each time I got a bolt from a nerve shock, I cringed. I felt like the devil had a Taser and he tased me, causing intense pain. *How long, God? How long will it be until life returns to normal?* Then doubt whispered, "Will I ever be normal again?"

Between the doubt, the pain, and the whispers from the enemy, a thought crossed my mind. I could end it all. I could be delivered into the arms of my Savior and free from all pain.

I brushed those temptations away, trying to be strong. Then one night, I couldn't move fast enough. I tried getting to the bathroom, but the pain slowed me down, and it wasn't pretty.

I felt humiliated as my husband cleaned up my mess. Let's just say he wasn't happy about it. Tears refused to stop, and I made the decision.

I crouched down by the sofa where Iva was lying. I hugged and kissed her black velvet nose, and through tears, I said goodbye.

Then I went to the kitchen, opened the cabinet door, and grabbed the first bottle of pills. I poured them into my hand. The bottle had recently been filled.

As I held those capsules in my palm, something happened. I couldn't do it. God stopped me. I lacked the courage to take my life, so I poured every pill back into the bottle and sat down with Iva.

Depression is a familiar foe to me, but I had never come that close to suicide. Looking back, I am glad God stopped me because I would have missed so much, and I would have ruined the testimony God has given me.

God's healing comes in His time, but I don't wait well. I anticipated the good God brought from this, and He did work it out for good. It's so hard holding on while we wait through horrible, unending trials.

The gospels of Matthew, Mark, and Luke tell us the story of the woman with the issue of blood. It clearly depicts her faith, but it also demonstrates her patience.

She had been hemorrhaging for twelve years without any help from doctors. She was poor after spending all her money on doctors. Many of them probably took advantage of her desire for healing.

There's no mention of a husband or family, which makes sense since anyone living with her would be ceremonially unclean because of her condition. She may have been quite lonely for the same reason.

She couldn't go to the temple to worship or find friends to encourage her. She couldn't have visits from her rabbi. Do you feel her loneliness and hopelessness?

Then she heard Jesus was in town, and she believed without a doubt that if she could just touch the hem of His garment, she would be healed. She planned to sneak into the crowd and accomplish this without being noticed.

It took all her strength to catch up to Jesus in the crowd surrounding Him, and she practically crawled between people as she stretched her skinny fingers to grasp His robe. Immediately she was healed, and Jesus knew it.

He didn't rebuke her. He lovingly encouraged her faith.

What are you waiting for: relief from pain, an appointment, or a diagnosis? During our trials, the enemy tempts us to doubt God. God takes that same trial and turns it into something good.

It took almost two years before I could see that, but I'm glad I waited on God.

Friend, I pray we don't have to wait as long as this woman, but I am with you in the waiting. While we wait, what do we do? I keep asking God, "What's the next thing?" That is all I can do.

What is the next thing for you? Don't get ahead of yourself. Just do the next thing.

Why are you cast down, O my soul?
And *why* are you disquieted within me?
Hope in God, for I shall yet praise Him
For the help of His countenance.
Psalm 42:5 NKJV

Heavenly Father, help me look toward the next thing and not get ahead of You. Comfort my heart when depression takes over and keep me far from the temptation of suicide. In Jesus's name. Amen.

Day 11

God's Sacred Design

I will praise You, for I am fearfully and wonderfully made;
Marvelous are Your works,
And *that* my soul knows very well.
Psalm 139:14 NKJV

"We can't do your surgery, so we're referring you to a deformity doctor."

I asked, "What kind of doctor?"

I couldn't believe what I just heard. Why did I need a deformity doctor? What was wrong with me? I didn't get those answers that day, but the doctor explained, "If we do the surgery, it will create issues, and you'll need a second surgery. This doctor can do all of it in one surgery."

I tried to remain calm as a flame of anger burned. I endured pain for almost four months, and finally someone decided to take a full back X-ray. Why didn't doctors do this earlier? Whatever they saw in this X-ray shed new light on my problem.

I understood the doctor's reluctance to operate. I didn't want two surgeries either, but disappointment flooded my heart.

I hated the word deformity. Even with my blindness, I had never been called deformed. Deformity sounded grotesque. I wanted to tell this doctor I am fearfully and wonderfully made by my Creator and Heavenly Father.

Tears ran freely when I got in the car. I sat in the front seat next to my husband, no longer needing to lie down in the back seat thanks to the epidurals. It went beyond the deformity thing. I had expected surgery in two weeks, so I could resume my life as normal by late January. Just when the finish line was in sight, someone moved it.

The doctor never told me what the deformity was. What horrible thing would I learn from a complex neurosurgeon?

Three weeks later, I learned something I already knew. I had scoliosis. Nobody had explained the severity of it to me until then. The neurosurgeon said, "Without a major surgery, your lungs and heart will be affected, and pain will increase."

God's creation is a masterpiece. We live in a sin-cursed world with sickness, which creates all sorts of havoc. "For we are God's masterpiece. He has created us anew in Christ Jesus, so we can do the good things he planned for us long ago" (Ephesians 2:10 NLT).

The Greek word translated masterpiece in the New Living Translation (NLT) is *poiēma*, and it means "beautiful poem." This same word is translated as workmanship in the New King James Version (NKJV).

Let's unpack our focal verse from Psalm 139:14. "Wonderfully made" means distinguished, and we are His marvelous works. Think about that. You are distinguished and marvelous.

I couldn't see the curvature of my spine, nor the twist in it on the X-ray, but after surgery, I saw my scars. I felt them, and I hated them. Scars ran up the middle of my back and stomach, measuring about eight to ten inches.

The spine surgery left me with an obvious abnormal bulge in my lower left abdomen. Even after a CAT scan, the doctors told me there was nothing there. It looked as if I was pregnant. I tried flattening it with tummy shapers. Whatever the nothing was, it eventually diminished.

I don't know about your scars, the ones you see and the internal ones you feel. I consider them battle trophies now. Is there something about your body that causes you unhappiness? You are a masterpiece, not a mess.

We began as beautiful poems and masterpieces, but sin has left its ugly mark on us. As women, we care about our appearances. But one day we will receive our glorified bodies. We will be perfect without deformities, scars, or pain.

Perhaps your scars are invisible, but you live in agonizing pain or sickness. Don't despise your body! It is the temple of the Holy Spirit.

Walk through these difficult days with grace, knowing you are more than your physical body. You are God's masterpiece.

> Or do you not know that your body is the temple of the Holy Spirit who is in you, whom you have from God, and you are not your own? For you were bought at a price; therefore glorify God in your body and in your spirit, which are God's.
> 1 Corinthians 6:19–20 NKJV

Heavenly Father, thank You for creating me as a masterpiece. Remove all feelings of dissatisfaction about my body. Help me glorify You in this body, with all its flaws. In Jesus's name. Amen.

Day 12

From Broken to Beautiful

"For I know the plans I have for you," declares the Lord,
"plans to prosper you and not to harm you,
plans to give you hope and a future."
Jeremiah 29:11 NIV

On the day I first encountered horrific pain, the Lord came to me. As I lay in the grass sobbing, He reminded me to rest, and then He tucked today's verse into my heart. The plans and future on my mind that day centered around marketing my new book. One by one, those plans went up in smoke, and only some ashes remained.

I couldn't handle the crippling pain of sciatica, and great discouragement surrounded me. All my speaker friends had events, but I had to cancel mine. I forgot the Lord's promise. My future looked bleak. I forgot about God's future and hope for me. *I am not a speaker. I'm finished.*

The epidurals helped the pain decrease, and life grew a bit brighter. I could attend church again, which brought me much needed joy. I also began walking Iva while using a cane. She adapted to the cane, and our walks grew a little longer each day. I had longed for this during the months I could barely walk. The Lord wrapped me in perfect peace concerning seeing the neurosurgeon and what we would learn on that visit.

My sweet friend, Pastor Edith, invited me to speak at her church. Could I do it? I still needed lots of medication, including pain meds, to function. Yes, with my overcomer attitude, I would do it!

I prepared the message, and the day arrived to speak. I had no idea how healing that day would be. I could never imagine the joy of boxing up books and driving down the interstate. God had brought me full circle. He restored me. He wasn't finished with me. His plans, His future, and His hope still existed.

I asked God to forgive me for doubting Him. Sometimes life takes us to hard places, where pain is relentless, and hope fades like the evening sun. We are flesh, but don't forget we have a Heavenly Father, and He has plans for a future and a hope. We give up on Him, but He never gives up on us.

Sadly, the doubts returned, and with them came discouragement. How quickly I forgot God's faithfulness. After surgery, I expected things to get better, not worse. Once again, I saw God's faithfulness.

God is in the restoration business. He heals. He restores family relationships. He restores loss. He restores marriages. He restores our health. Most importantly, He restores our hope.

When Jeremiah penned these words, he wrote to Jewish exiles in Babylon. They had lost all hope. As captives, all they had left were their lives and possibly some personal items.

God wanted His people to hang onto hope because their captivity would last seventy years. He wants us to hang onto hope in the same manner. He promised, "I will repay you for the years the locusts have eaten—the great locust and the young locust" (Joel 2:25 NIV).

We cannot understand God's ways, but we must trust Him. When God has another plan, it will be better than anything we can imagine (Ephesians 3:20). Why can't we trust God to turn it around?

God makes beauty from brokenness. God takes the broken parts of our hearts, our relationships, our bank accounts, and our health, and He works them all together, like a baker kneading bread. Then He makes something beautiful from all the broken parts, and it is His plan and purpose for our lives.

My friend, right now, it looks like all is lost. Have you forgotten the promises of God? Do you feel overlooked? Do you think life will never be the same?

I want to squeeze your hand and whisper this gentle reminder. God hasn't abandoned you. He still has that purpose and future for you. He still has hopes and plans for you.

What promise can you cling to today? How can you trust God for a future and a plan?

> And we know that in all things God works for
> the good of those who love him, who have been
> called according to his purpose.
> Romans 8:28 NIV

Father God, help me realize You restore broken lives. Like a carpenter bringing new life to an old piece of furniture, You are at work, and I don't even know it. Help me trust You to do the supernatural, the unexpected, and the miraculous. In Jesus's name. Amen.

Day 13

Should I Have This Surgery?

Your ears shall hear a word behind you, saying,
"This *is* the way, walk in it,"
Whenever you turn to the right hand
Or whenever you turn to the left.
Isaiah 30:21 NKJV

Surgeons planned to drill two rods and eighteen screws into my back. The doctor told me that my hospital stay could last six days, and the recovery would take months. I'd have to wear a back brace for a long time. The neurosurgeon kept telling me that this was a major surgery. But I'd never had many surgeries, so I didn't grasp his definition of a major surgery. The first thing I realized while sitting in his office was that I would have to step away from ministry. I would have to put all my energy into healing. I still had no clue what I faced.

Timmy explained the severity of my scoliosis. "Your spine looks like it is pregnant," he explained as he traced out a huge bulge on my back.

The prognosis sounded great. No chance of death or paralysis. It would correct all my problems and pain.

I searched for "spinal fusion" online. I refrained from watching the videos about risks or bad results. My neurosurgeon warned me about several complications: pneumonia, blood clots, infection, and blood loss.

I had to wait over three months to have surgery and live with pain longer than I wanted. I used that time to prepare myself spiritually. A few weeks prior to surgery, I began having second thoughts. At the doctor's office, I felt peaceful. During the first couple of months, I remained at peace, but now I wondered if I should have this major spinal fusion. I was doing fine by taking the meds. The pain wasn't as bad as it once was. *Do I really want to live on all this medication? Don't I want to be free from pain?*

I'm still part of a spinal fusion Facebook group. Whenever I read a post from someone asking if they should have surgery, I never comment. Only God can tell you if you should have surgery. Spinal fusions can vary depending on how many vertebrae they fuse.

God guides us through big decisions. No, the answers don't show up on a billboard, but they are printed on our hearts. It takes prayer and patience. We don't necessarily get answers as quickly as David when He inquired of the Lord as to whether he should fight the Philistines (2 Samuel 5:19). I don't recommend putting out a fleece like Gideon did in Judges 6, but I prefer several confirmations to make sure I am hearing the Lord correctly.

James instructs us under the inspiration of the Holy Spirit to ask God for wisdom (James 1:5). He says God will give wisdom liberally.

Seeking God's counsel is also part of abiding in Christ. Jesus said we can do nothing apart from Him (John 15:4).

How do we know when we have God's answer? He will give us peace that passes all understanding. I learned this from a dear woman of God many years ago when my husband needed a bone marrow transplant to live. He had no peace about the transplant and refused to have it. Panic filled me while I tried to support him. Then a new door opened suddenly. A clinical trial was producing remarkable results for people with the same leukemia he had. Patients were going into remission. He's still alive twenty-five years later thanks to God.

Friend, are you struggling to decide about surgery? Are you fighting with insurance to cover a much-needed treatment? We've done that too. God opens the right doors at the right time, while locking all other doors. He has plans for us. He knew about that clinical trial long before scientists did. He knew, many years ago before my spine began curving, that I would need this major surgery. He knows what you need.

Spend time with the Lord. Get in His Word and pray. Seek His face, and He will direct your paths.

And the peace of God,
which surpasses all understanding,
will guard your hearts
and minds through Christ Jesus.
Philippians 4:7 NKJV

Heavenly Father, surgery is scary, but You have gifted surgeons with skills that fuse lives back together. I seek Your wisdom. Please show me the door You want me to walk through. Shut and bolt all other doors so I will not enter them. In Jesus's name. Amen.

Day 14

Seeking Comfort

Praise be to the God and Father of our Lord Jesus Christ, the Father of compassion and the God of all comfort, who comforts us in all our troubles, so that we can comfort those in any trouble with the comfort we ourselves receive from God.
2 Corinthians 1:3–4 NIV

After seven hours of surgery, a nurse woke me up in the recovery room. My friend stayed with me while they moved me to my hospital room and until Timmy arrived. He had gone home during the lengthy surgery.

With sixty-two staples in my back, a huge incision in my abdomen, and drains and wires going everywhere, I tried to find a comfortable position, but it proved impossible. I tried lying on my right side, but that didn't last long. Then I rolled onto my back with the nurses' help, but that also created pain. I tried my left side and discovered no matter which position I tried, no comfort could be found.

The next day, a physical therapist showed me how to put on the heavy back brace filled with metal and Velcro, and I had to wear it every time I was out of bed. I had a surprise visit from some church friends and a beautiful vase of flowers from one of my speaker groups.

After three days, they sent me home, and I couldn't wait to sleep in my own bed, but I still couldn't find comfort. The church set up a meal train, so I had a flow of visitors and phone calls. Many of these people had traversed their own seasons of suffering, and they empathized with me.

My body found no comfort, but God covered me with His loving comfort like a warm blanket. Hospitals offer warm blankets, and while the blanket doesn't fix the problem, it does make us feel better.

God's compassion comforts our spirits when our bodies hurt. He comes alongside us to comfort us in our suffering. He comforts us, so we can comfort others.

God allows our suffering, although He doesn't cause our suffering. Even though our pain is health related and not caused by religious persecution, it is still considered the sufferings of Jesus Christ. "For just as we share abundantly in the sufferings of Christ, so also our comfort abounds through Christ" (2 Corinthians 1:5 NIV).

This verse shows us that, although God allows the suffering, He brings the comfort. He doesn't want us to be comfortless. We also learn from this passage that after we navigate suffering, we can help and offer comfort to others.

We receive that comfort through the lovely fragrance of the flowers someone sends, the greeting cards that trickle in, and the concerned visitors who come by to pray with us. Comfort also shows up in phone calls, text messages, and even through the home health workers.

I see this portrait of love more clearly now in retrospect. I know I was truly blessed, and I hope you receive that same compassion. Sadly, I know sometimes people suffer alone. That's not God's plan, because He wants us to comfort others with the same comfort we have received.

Where does your comfort come from? Since you are reading this book, I hope it is a source of comfort to you, especially if you are alone. I want to take the horrible season of suffering I endured and share it with encouragement. I want to shed light into your mysterious world. I want to share the Bible verses I discovered along the way that I had never noticed before.

One day, my friend, you will extend comfort to someone in need. How can you lean into God as a compassionate comforter? God comforts us with the comfort that is greater than all others. Meditate on this verse:

> If we are distressed, it is for your comfort
> and salvation; if we are comforted, it is for
> your comfort, which produces in you patient
> endurance of the same sufferings we suffer.
> (2 Corinthians 1:6 NIV)

One day, you will recognize this same patient endurance Paul wrote about above as you share comfort with someone else.

God of all comfort, thank You for the comfort You bestow on me. Thank You for Your love and mercy. Though I may be alone, I am never alone with You, Father God. In Jesus's name. Amen.

Day 15

Trusting God Through the Silence

I cry out to you, God, but you do not answer;
I stand up, but you merely look at me.
Job 30:20 NIV

Have you felt alone in your suffering? No one understands it, not family or friends. They send messages thinking you are on the mend when that couldn't be further from the truth. They wonder why they don't see you at church or the grocery store. They don't have a clue about your suffering, and worst of all, even God is silent.

I felt alone because each night after my spinal fusion surgery was a repeat of the night before. The pain never ceased, and I couldn't get comfortable in bed, no matter how many pillows Timmy tucked around me. The recliner helped at times, but often pain continued throughout the night. No answer to prayers came. No word or Scripture was heard. Hope faded like a late summer bloom, and peace vanished like steam off a cup of hot chocolate. Pain replaced peace.

I slept some during the afternoons, but both of us felt exhausted from my inability to rest due to pain.

I couldn't bend, so I needed help dressing, and now I needed to wear Depends because some of my body's nerves had gone numb during the surgery, preventing me from knowing when I had to go to the bathroom. Thankfully, this problem didn't last long, but one night, due to weariness, we both fell asleep without getting my new underwear on, and I woke up in a puddle.

I felt like I was living in a nightmare, and I just wanted to wake up and find out it was over, but when I awoke, it was quite real. Can you relate, sweet friend?

You've been in that nightmare too. Meds aren't helping. The heating pad or ice pack proves useless. Mental anguish goes with your physical suffering. You toss and turn, if you're able, but sleep evades you. Relief refuses to come, and in all this God remains silent.

In all his sufferings, Job felt like us, sweet friend. We're not alone in our feelings of abandonment.

In a matter of hours, Job lost everything: his children, his livestock, and his servants. Mrs. Job wasn't much help when she told Job to curse God and die. Then Job was covered in painful boils. "Days of suffering grip me. Night pierces my bones; my gnawing pains never rest" (Job 30:16–17 NIV).

Can you relate to Job as much as I can? It helps to know I am not alone, and that may comfort you also. Someone else understands us.

I stopped hoping that beauty would arise out of those ashes. Job seemed to share those same doubts. "I am reduced to dust and ashes" (Job 30:19 NIV). Would life ever return to normal? How much of this would end, and what would I have to live with forever?

Job said, "Yet when I hoped for good, evil came; when I looked for light, then came darkness. The churning inside me never stops; days of suffering confront me" (Job 30:26–27 NIV).

Does this sound familiar, friend? Well, I have good news. Job survived. I survived, and you will survive too. When God is silent, it doesn't mean the answer is no. He works on our behalf in the background without a word to us.

There's someone else who knows how you feel besides Job and me. Jesus Christ experienced pain, suffering, rejection, and anguish on this earth. Although He may be silent, He knows how you feel. He has compassion and mercy for you. He hates seeing the effects sin has had on this earth, including sickness and pain.

Can you hang on to that today? Can that truth be the light in your darkness? Hold on tight, because tonight, you may forget.

Write it down so you'll see it and recall it. Jesus knows. Jesus cares, and He is working on your behalf.

Because of the Lord's great love
we are not consumed,
for his compassions never fail.
They are new every morning;
great is your faithfulness.
Lamentations 3:22–23 NIV

Jesus, You know how I feel, because You have felt tremendous pain. You endured it all for me, and You would have endured it all for just me. Please bring an end to my pain and heal me! In Your name I pray. Amen.

Day 16

Reclaiming Peace

Do not be anxious about anything, but in every
situation, by prayer and petition, with thanksgiving,
present your requests to God. And the peace of God,
which transcends all understanding, will guard
your hearts and your minds in Christ Jesus.
Philippians 4:6–7 NIV

I turned my walker around at the end of my driveway. The summer sun made my heavy, black back brace feel like a sauna. Birds sang perched in the branches of the tree above me that shaded our driveway. Why couldn't I find any pleasure on a beautiful summer evening? I breathed in the aroma of flowers, but I still felt empty.

Then I realized I had allowed the post-surgical pain and complications to steal my peace and joy. My faith had wavered, leaving me feeling hopeless. A bolt of anger made me determined to take back what the enemy had stolen. As I walked my laps to strengthen my body, I drew strength from the Holy Spirit. Then I recalled our focal verses, and I knew what to do. God gives us a remedy for peace if we are willing to take it.

First, stop being anxious. Don't worry. I couldn't ignore my body's cry for relief, but I didn't need to make it my focus. That's the place for Jesus. I gave in to thoughts of discouragement instead of taking thoughts captive. I focused on the sleepless nights and debilitating pain. Even during constant pain, I could count my blessings if I chose to do so. We must consciously remove discouraging thoughts. Stop worrying about why God hasn't healed us, and concentrate on every blessing.

Worry makes us step into a role we were never created to fill. As children, we didn't worry about having food on the table or keeping the house warm in winter. In some cases, children have those worries, but most of us trusted our parents to provide for us.

God is greater than any earthly father. He is Jehovah Jireh, our provider. Worry says we can't trust our Father to provide. Worry says we are trying to be the parent and not the child.

Next, I needed to depend on God even though He hadn't answered my pleas for relief. I could pray more often with more faith. I could trust Him in the dark. I could spend less time complaining.

Finally, give thanks. God commands thankfulness because gratitude benefits us immensely. It sets our minds on a new track. We begin thinking with a positive outlook rather than a negative one. Isn't it easy to fall into thoughts of what we lack rather than count our blessings?

I thanked God for many things once I stopped the stinking thinking, the negative thoughts I entertained. I could walk! I didn't have pneumonia or blood clots, which were potential complications. My wonderful husband took care of me. I had my beautiful guide dog, Iva, by my side, even as I did laps in the driveway. She insisted on being with me.

Our circumstances cannot give us joy, peace, or hope. Why do we lose those precious gifts when things go wrong? Joy only comes from Jesus. He is our joy and our peace, and He is our only hope.

When we stop the anxious thoughts and pray with thankful hearts, God promises us a peace that is beyond comprehension. He promises to guard our hearts and minds with His peace. He will guard them against anxiety, discouragement, and doubt.

The word guard is a military term. God is setting troops of holy soldiers around our hearts and minds.

I know your circumstances are daunting, but we can't allow the enemy to steal what Jesus has given us. Find Scriptures to help you focus on joy and hope. Stop the anxiety. Pray more and give God thanks, and peace will return. What you are enduring is so hard. Don't give in to what you go through.

What will you allow to occupy your mind? In the following verse, the word let means to allow. Allow God's peace and not the devil's panic to rule your heart.

And let the peace of God rule in your hearts, to
which also you were called in one body;
and be thankful.
Colossians 3:15 NKJV

Lord Jesus, help me resist the urge to give in to worry. Thank You for being my one hope. Life is rough right now, but I know You have a plan, and I need to wait on You. In Your name I pray. Amen.

Day 17

Patience in His Purpose

Wait on the Lord;
Be of good courage,
And He shall strengthen your heart;
Wait, I say, on the Lord!
Psalm 27:14 NKJV

October's colorful leaves marked five months since surgery, which changed my life. I was still waiting ... waiting for spinal healing, waiting for my energy to return, waiting for my nerves to repair, and waiting for doors in my ministry to open.

I was also still waiting for my life to become normal again, and I wondered if it ever would. I continually prayed for these things, and I wanted to believe they would happen.

As this verse popped out at me, I realized something. I was waiting on what I wanted God to do. I wasn't waiting for Him to do what He wanted to do. Perhaps healing needed to take longer. Maybe ministry opportunities would come in a different form. Ever since this painful journey began over a year earlier,

I'd been learning to submit to God's will, not Carolyn's. That's a difficult thing to do.

Let's unpack this verse. When we wait on the Lord, we must have an active obedience. As I said earlier, I was waiting for what I thought should happen. We must understand we might be waiting for something quite different than what we expect. If we don't open our hearts to God's will, we might miss His perfect plans for us.

I have to remind myself when I pray that I must put God's purposes before my own. I must be open to the changes God may have in store for me.

Be of good courage! We must possess an active faith during our waiting. How many times do we lose faith and hope while waiting? The past year was filled with hopelessness and faithlessness for me. Unbearable pain and complications pushed me off my firm foundation. An active and living faith helps us wait.

When we trust confidently in the Lord, He will also strengthen our hearts. He will meet us in our desire to keep faith alive while we wait. God wants our faith to become stronger, not fall apart.

In the Christian life, we wait while we work. We aren't seated in a waiting room. We're not placed on hold listening to elevator music. Waiting isn't a time to be passive, but active. We can't be active about the thing we are waiting for, but there's something else we can do in the meantime. A lot can be written about what happens in the meantime.

God may have detours for us that take us down roads we would have never traveled except for this journey of waiting. He may have stops for us to make that we would have never considered. We must be open to these changes.

Are you waiting? I'm not going to ask you what you are waiting for. That would imply what you want to happen. You are waiting on God's answer to your problem. Don't miss His answer with selective vision.

Wait with an active faith. Encourage yourself in the Word daily. Ask God to strengthen your heart. He promises here that He will.

Wait with activity. You are in the meantime, the time when much transpires. Get busy with whatever God directs you to do in the meantime.

The enemy will attack us with doubt in seasons of waiting. He dangles ideas that we latch onto. These can interfere with our waiting. Sweet friend, please don't allow doubt to rock your faith nor give place to the devil (Ephesians 4:27).

We give the devil opportunities to shatter our faith, filling us with doubt. This leads to discouragement, disappointment, and even depression. It also grieves the Holy Spirit, and I found myself in that situation.

It's no coincidence we find the command about grieving the Holy Spirit just three verses later. When we give the enemy a place, we grieve the Spirit.

How can you wait without giving the enemy a place and grieving the Spirit? Dear friend, if you feel you've already done that, it's never too late. Begin by abiding in Christ. That is the perfect place to wait.

And do not grieve the Holy Spirit of God,
by whom you were sealed for the day of
redemption.
Ephesians 4:30 NKJV

Lord Jesus, I long to abide in You. Keep me from falling for the enemy's deception. In Your name I pray. Amen.

Day 18

Beyond the Storm

Looking unto Jesus, the author and finisher of our faith,
who for the joy that was set before Him endured the cross,
despising the shame, and has sat down at the right
hand of the throne of God.
Hebrews 12:2 NKJV

I no longer needed pain medication, but I needed medicine to help with neuropathy and restless leg syndrome. My blood work indicated I was low in several things, so my doctor prescribed some more medications. I hated taking all these meds because they usually caused some side effects.

The days grew shorter, and I wondered if I was experiencing Seasonal Affective Disorder (SAD), which is understandable since I don't see much light due to my blindness.

I struggled that winter with weather-related pain, tingling feet, and running legs. My numb leg couldn't get warm. I tried a heating pad, but my nerves couldn't detect the heat.

Mornings were enjoyable with prayer, Bible study, and walks with Iva, but by afternoon, I fell into a slump. I couldn't shake the feeling that something just wasn't right with my body. I felt depressed, but not the lows I had experienced before.

One of my new medications created feelings of anxiety and depression. After my doctor changed that medication, I immediately felt better.

Pain and illness demand our attention. It's hard to ignore because it invades every part of our lives. I couldn't take my mind off the torment I felt.

We must focus on God instead of our suffering. In Matthew 14, Jesus sent His disciples across a calm sea in a boat. When they reached the middle of the Sea of Galilee, they grew weary trying to row against the churning waves and strong winds. These were seasoned fishermen, but this fierce storm frightened them.

Jesus walked across the stormy sea to His terrified disciples. At first, they grew even more afraid, because they didn't recognize Him, but He called out to them. Filled with boldness, Peter requested to walk with Jesus on the water. Peter climbed out of the boat and walked across the waves until he saw that the wind was boisterous (Matthew 14:30). The strong gusts churned the water like a mixer.

Peter began to sink. He had taken his eyes off Jesus and put his focus on the storm.

Pain and physical afflictions were the boisterous winds that took my eyes off Jesus. Like Peter, I sank into a sea with waves of discouragement.

What are the boisterous winds in your life that steal your focus from Jesus? When we look at the heartache, our faith weakens. We look at the dwindling bank account. We look at the pain and sickness. We look at the things we can no longer do because our bodies don't allow it.

When our eyes aren't on Jesus, our faith loses power. We begin to sink. For us, this can occur over days, weeks, and even months, but for Peter, it happened in just a few seconds.

Moments might have seemed like hours as Peter wondered why Jesus allowed him to sink. Where was the boldness he had only one minute earlier?

Peter cried out to Jesus, "Lord, save me!" (Matthew 14:30 NIV). It's in the sinking that we realign our focus and our faith. Moments of sinking become moments of strengthening. Where did Peter place his focus when he cried out to Jesus? He focused on Christ. He also had enough faith to know Jesus would rescue him.

Are you sinking in a sea of hopelessness? That's where I found myself, and I must admit, it took me a while to realign my focus. I was treading water for a while. If you find yourself in that stormy water today, this is your time for a realignment. Set your eyes on Jesus. Focus on Christ, not the crisis. Friend, He will rescue you, just like He rescued Peter. Don't keep depending on your own strength to tread water. Realign your focus. Realign your faith. Trust His strength to fight against the strong storms in your life.

Abide in Me, and I in you.
As the branch cannot bear fruit of itself,
unless it abides in the vine, neither can you,
unless you abide in Me.
John 15:4 NKJV

Heavenly Father, I need to realign my focus and my faith. Forgive me for allowing life to distract me, but I need a rescue right now. Walk with me through this storm, and I will continually stare into Your face, knowing You hold me. In Jesus's name. Amen.

Day 19

Guard Your Mind

And do not be conformed to this world, but be transformed by the renewing of your mind, that you may prove what *is* that good and acceptable and perfect will of God.
Romans 12:2 NKJV

The promise of a new day greeted me after a night of wrestling with restless leg syndrome. I tried to walk a little farther. I pushed myself to do some light housework, then I felt drained. I should have had more strength than this by that time in my recovery.

Darkness and depression surrounded me. I lacked any desire to do anything, and I forced myself to accomplish each task. I used to love writing. Why was it so difficult?

That's when a nap and binge watching some crime dramas sounded like a plan. Sleep didn't come, but thoughts invaded my mind. *Life as you knew it is over. Why serve a God who allows this? Your ministry is done.*

Amid thoughts and dozing off, I had a vision. I saw myself on a stage speaking to a large crowd. This vision returned continually.

Don't allow physical limitations to become mental limitations. The enemy sows seeds of doubt and discouragement in our minds. He filled the heart of Ananias to lie about the price of his land to the Holy Spirit (Acts 5:3).

It's easier to take thoughts captive than to pull down strongholds. Left to take root in our minds, these anxious thoughts become strongholds. This is why we must renew our minds daily.

How do we renew our minds? Act like a guard over your mind and seize those troublesome thoughts immediately. Think on things that are pure, lovely, and noble (Philippians 4:8). Think on things above and not on this earth (Colossians 3:2).

Don't just read the Word of God, but meditate on it. Select a verse and roll it over in your mind throughout the day. Pray through the Scriptures and pray often.

Pain and sickness can draw us away from our Bibles and prayer. This is when we need the mind of Christ. "For God has not given us a spirit of fear, but of power and of love and of a sound mind" (2 Timothy 1:7 NKJV).

Fearful thoughts often settle in our minds during seasons of physical suffering. We see in this verse that these thoughts don't come from God. They come from the enemy or our flesh, but God gives us a sound mind. Christ gave us victory in His death and resurrection. We need to stand in that victory. We need to keep our minds sound and prevent them from being polluted with thoughts that lead to anxiety and depression.

We also need to keep a spiritual mind. We are filled with the Holy Spirit, and His power flows through us, even when we feel weak. The Word of God will fuel that power, and with that power, we can reject the fears the enemy taunts us with.

Then there is love. Perfect love casts out fear (1 John 4:18). We have nothing to fear because Christ conquered it all with His death on the cross. His perfect love provided us with the way to salvation.

Living with pain and chronic illness with no visible change in sight gives us reason to fret. This is our physical well-being we're talking about. The commands that say don't fear and don't worry are woven throughout Scripture, but when it comes to our health, it becomes difficult to do.

Before I faced these trials, I believed I could not have faith while I was fearful. Fear is a fiery arrow shot by the enemy to destroy our faith. It damaged my faith, but God is faithful and gives us resilient faith.

As we renew our minds, we will put out these fires of fear. Our minds and hearts are fragile, but the peace of God guards them (Philippians 4:7).

A renewed mind will crush fear. A stable heart will shield us from worry. Faith isn't the absence of fear. It's the presence of God.

Sweet friend, what steps can you take to renew your mind today? Will you linger in the Word and prayer?

What fears are you wrestling with today? How can God's Word help you quench the fiery arrows of fear?

For "who has known the mind of the Lord that
he may instruct Him?"
But we have the mind of Christ.
1 Corinthians 2:16 NKJV

Heavenly Father, so many deceptive thoughts bombard my mind. Put a guard over my mind and reveal the truth I need to believe and live out. In Jesus's name. Amen.

Day 20

A New Perspective

We are afflicted in every way but not crushed;
we are perplexed but not in despair;
we are persecuted but not abandoned;
we are struck down but not destroyed.
2 Corinthians 4:8–9 CSB

Some nights, I lay awake, unable to find comfort with all the metal in my back. People ask me, "Can you feel the metal?" I don't feel the rods and screws themselves, but I do feel this incredible heaviness I never had before, a constraint from the fusion that limits my movement. The pain intensifies in the cold.

One night, my legs wanted to run a marathon, while I wanted to sleep. Snow continued falling, and forecasters expected bitter cold breezes, limiting my activity outside and increasing my pain. I missed walking because the more I walked, the less I hurt. Sadly, the weather hindered the one thing that offered me some relief.

I remember seasons of depression when emotional pain kept me awake too. Many times, anxiety accompanies chronic pain and illness. It feels like you fight three battles: the physical, emotional, and spiritual.

Honestly, I grow quite discontented in my discomfort, and I don't like that. I need a new attitude.

Pain afflicts me, but it doesn't control me. When I'm tempted to sink into despair, I find strength by remembering the words of Paul. He endured stoning, beatings, shipwreck, and imprisonment. Yet, he wrote the verses above in a chapter where he uses lots of contrasts to help his readers understand that the sufferings of this world are a momentary light affliction compared to the eternal weight of glory we will receive (2 Corinthians 4:17).

When I try to look at my suffering as a momentary light affliction, I can agree with Paul in our focal verses. Paul's words remind me I am not the first to feel this way, and I am not alone in it. I'm changing my perspective. As we unpack these verses, I'm using the Amplified Bible to shed more light on the meaning.

"We are pressured in every way [hedged in], but not crushed" (2 Corinthians 4:8 AMP). Paul was pressured in every way but not crushed. We know that pressure: health, finances, and family pressures, but like Paul, we're still standing. Even when I feel squeezed by life, I can find blessings when I give thanks.

"Perplexed [unsure of finding a way out], but not driven to despair" (2 Corinthians 4:8 AMP). I must admit I have allowed my complications to drive me to despair, but I don't have to visit that dark place, and neither do you. We can ask Jesus to heal us and not lose hope. We can grow in His grace and mercy. We can trust His sovereign will. We can move forward in our situation with His all-sufficient grace.

"Hunted down and persecuted, but not deserted [to stand alone]" (2 Corinthians 4:9 AMP). We can face persecution, and Jesus never forsakes us. He doesn't abandon us in our pain either. He doesn't abandon us in our discouragement. Even when He hasn't answered our prayers, and disappointment drops in, He will never leave us.

"Struck down, but never destroyed" (2 Corinthians 4:9 AMP). We can be struck down, but we are not destroyed. We'll never be destroyed because of Christ. Even death cannot destroy the child of God.

Instead of stewing in my pain, I want to soak in the Scriptures. I am not crushed, not in despair, never forsaken or destroyed. I repeat the words until I feel peace and sleep finds me.

Many of you suffer through pain much worse than I do, and you probably handle it better. When pain presses in, how might God use this Scripture to steady your heart? What would it look like to speak these truths over your hardest moments?

Whatever battle you face today, you are never abandoned, and you are not without hope. Find encouragement in these instructions to Joshua.

> Have I not commanded you? Be strong and of
> good courage; do not be afraid,
> nor be dismayed, for the Lord your God *is* with
> you wherever you go."
> Joshua 1:9 NKJV

Heavenly Father, help me remember You have a glorious home awaiting me, and what I suffer through today will appear small when compared to the glory that awaits me. Help me through these days. I need healing, grace, and mercy. Help me rest and give You glory from my suffering. In Jesus's name. Amen.

Day 21

Going in the Strength of the Lord

I will go in the strength of the Lord God;
I will make mention of Your righteousness, of Yours only.
Psalm 71:16 NKJV

Weariness overwhelmed me. Muscle aches tempted me because all I wanted to do was rest, but I had too much to do. I prayed while reading my Bible. This verse spoke to me like a good medicine. I sought strength from my Lord because mine had dissipated.

Elijah went in the strength of the Lord. He hosted a showdown with the 450 false prophets of Baal (1 Kings 18:22). Their false god didn't send fire down on their altar, but God rained fire down on Elijah's sacrifice. Elijah slaughtered all the false prophets.

Next, Elijah fervently prayed for the rain God had promised after their three-and-a-half-year drought. Then, like the Energizer Bunny, Elijah just kept going by outrunning King Ahab to Jezreel (1 Kings 18:46).

That's when things changed. You've had those days when everything's going great, and suddenly, something goes wrong. Elijah learned that despite his Mount Carmel victory and the much-needed downpour, evil Queen Jezebel wanted to kill him for taking the lives of her beloved false prophets. Once again, Elijah ran until he could go no farther, but now he ran in fear.

Jezebel sent a messenger with her threat, but why didn't she send an assassin to do the job instead of just a messenger? Our enemy sends threats to us because God won't allow him to send out the assassin. It still gets results because we fail to resist the threat. We respond rather than resist.

Don't give in to what you go through. This is difficult to do, but resist the disappointment. Resist the discouragement. Resist the what ifs that flood your mind. Resist the devil, and he will flee (James 4:7). Friend, aren't you glad to know someone like Elijah has failed to resist the threat, just like we do?

Jesus has already won our battle. We must stand firm on His victory. We cannot give up the hope, peace, and joy Christ has given us. When we fail to resist, we lose ground. Every time the enemy sends you a threat, resist him.

Elijah prayed for God to take his life, and he finally slept. When Elijah awoke, an angel served him food and water (1 Kings 19:5). The angel told Elijah to eat, drink, and rest some more.

Friend, we aren't running marathons or wiping out modern-day false prophets, but we get weak. We grow tired. We must go when we don't feel like going. Can you relate?

God wants us to rest because it's vital for life. Notice God's compassion as He cared for Elijah's physical needs with sleep, food, and water. Can you recall a time when God ministered to your physical needs?

Sometimes, we must push forward in the strength of the Lord (not overworking and foolishly going without rest). On the days when things must be done, trust in the Lord's strength.

Elijah battled depression after his biggest spiritual victory. I've struggled with it myself. Trust me, when we are under the dark cloud of depression, we must go in the strength of the Lord. Depression sucks up our energy like a vacuum cleaner snatching up crumbs.

Stress can also be a culprit. Carrying a heavy load wears us down. It affects us mentally, physically, and even spiritually. If you find yourself there today, ask the Lord for His strength. God brought comfort to Elijah, and Jezebel never killed him. Someone killed her, and Elijah went to heaven in a chariot of fire.

Paul said it best: "For when I am weak, then I am strong" (2 Corinthians 12:10 NKJV). God wants us to depend on Him. God doesn't want super-powerful children. He wants children who are super-infused with His power.

What must you accomplish today? Seek God's strength for that activity. Are you getting the rest and physical nourishment you need? How can you rely on God's strength?

Give God the glory for those areas of weakness because that's where His power shines bright. Let God show up and show off.

Heavenly Father, I'm glad I can be myself in Your presence. Broken and weak. My strength is faulty at best. Strengthen me physically and especially spiritually. I need Your Holy Spirit's power. In Jesus's name. Amen.

Day 22

The Sweet Spot in My Pain

I want to know Christ—
yes, to know the power of his resurrection and participation in his sufferings, becoming like him in his death.
Philippians 3:10 NIV

When I tried to pray, words escaped me. All that flowed from my mouth was, "Help me, Lord!" Mornings were the worst. Gone were the days of bouncing out of bed, feeding Iva, and going for our walks.

Now getting out of bed exhausted me. With each determined step, pain tempted me to give up, but I had to get better. I had to keep moving, so life could be normal again. After a few slow, painful laps down the hallway and through the kitchen, I worked the stiffness out.

After the surgery, walking became easier. Getting in and out of bed remained problematic, especially while keeping my back perfectly straight. I feared any wrong move might mess up the hardware in my back.

On my hardest days, I thought about the crown of thorns piercing the head of my Savior as blood trickled down His face. I couldn't imagine the severity of His pain. I thought about the deep agony He endured as men hammered wooden spikes into His hands and feet. He withstood all that pain for me and you, my friend.

Many times, I turned to distractions during the worst hours of my pain. If the Hallmark Channel didn't have a good Christmas movie on, I read. I found myself reading the bestseller of all time most often, the Bible. What better words to read to take my mind off the horrific pain.

Pain is an invitation to draw closer to Christ. As I landed on today's focal verse, I meditated on it for a while, then I studied it deeper.

"I want to know Christ." Don't hurry past this statement. It doesn't mean to gain more head knowledge about Christ. The Greek word for "know" implies an experiential knowledge. It's the kind of knowledge that comes from spending time with Christ. It means we must hang out with Him.

We want "to know the power of His resurrection." When God saved us, the Holy Spirit immediately took up residence within us. We have Christ's resurrection power living within us through the power of the Holy Spirit. Christ brought us from death to life. We were dead in our sins, but now we live because Christ lives.

Are we "participating in His sufferings"? I paused on this line. I'm suffering, but not to the extent Christ suffered. My pain cannot compare to what Christ endured as they beat Him, plucked His beard, then nailed Him to a cross to die a cruel death.

How do we participate in His sufferings? While we live in the agony of physical or emotional pain, Christ draws closer to us. Until we walk through pain, we will not know these gifts of comfort Christ gives us.

While He draws me to Himself, I feel His closeness. I learn to lean on Him in ways I never could apart from suffering. I see His miracles, and I know Him in a deeper sense all because of pain.

Am I "becoming like Him in His death"? One day, we will see Christ face-to-face. We will receive glorified bodies free from pain and disease. We will be resurrected from the dead when Christ takes us to our forever home. Doesn't that make you want to shout, "Hallelujah"?

Friend, we don't want to hurt, physically or emotionally. If you are suffering, how can you draw closer to Christ during this unique time? This is the sweet spot in our suffering. Our confidence is in Christ. For a strong faith, we must *know* Him, *know* the power of His resurrection, participate in His sufferings, and one day, wake up in His likeness.

Suffering invites unique blessings we'd never see except through pain. While on this earth, Christ knew extreme pain, and that's why He can relate to us while we suffer.

For we do not have a high priest who is unable
to empathize with our weaknesses, but we have
one who has been tempted in every way, just as
we are—yet he did not sin.
Hebrews 4:15 NIV

Lord Jesus, thank You for experiencing pain and suffering. You felt it while You lived here and especially at Your death. Through pain, I can come to know You even more. In Your name I pray. Amen.

Day 23

Finding Strength When You're Down

I have set the Lord always before me;
Because *He is* at my right hand I shall not be moved.
Therefore my heart is glad, and my glory rejoices;
My flesh also will rest in hope.
Psalm 16: 8–9 NKJV

It felt like I was falling in slow motion, and the fear of messing up my hardware consumed me. I skidded on the asphalt and ripped my jeans. How could a beautiful November morning walk with Iva change so quickly?

I sat up, then I realized I didn't know how to stand up without something to push off of, and I wasn't going to use Iva for that purpose.

No one was outside in our quiet neighborhood, so I called my husband. No answer. Next, I called my neighbor, "I fell while walking, and I'm on Linden."

"Oh, honey, we're on vacation. Can you call the rescue squad?"

"Okay. Bye."

I had no intention of calling 911 to tell them I'd fallen, and I couldn't get up. I didn't know what damage I had done to my back, if any. I tried reaching my husband again, and as I talked to him, a police car pulled up. My neighbor had made the call for me.

Someone helped me up, and I experienced no back pain, just a bloody knee. My doctor prescribed another round of physical therapy for balance and strengthening exercises, and that's where I learned how to stand up after a fall.

A deeper problem remained that physical therapy could not address. Discouragement left me emotionally down, and I lacked the strength to pull myself up and out of the darkness I was living in.

Jesus is the light of the world, and He doesn't want us living in darkness, not just the darkness of sin, but the darkness that accompanies emotional trauma. Our bodies cry out for relief and healing. When it doesn't come, we feel dejected. We allow our feelings to rule our thoughts.

How do we find the strength to pull ourselves up when we are down? In our focal verse, the psalmist says he has set the Lord always before him. I struggled to keep my eyes on Jesus while despondency wrapped its tentacles around me. The answer to my prayers was "No" and "Wait."

In our deepest anguish, we must keep Jesus at the center of our thoughts. Never give up! Notice the psalmist says always, not just when life is great, but all the time, and especially in the tough times.

When we put our eyes on Jesus, our flesh will rest in hope, as opposed to resting in the darkness of anxiety. That isn't the true rest we need. Hope will fill our souls, and it will reach our flesh. We begin by believing we have hope, because we do, no matter how hopeless we feel. We choose to hold onto hope, and it will go beyond our spirit and soul, touching our flesh. Hope is the lifeline that pulls us out of discouragement. As we focus on God and hold onto hope, we will find joy.

"You will show me the path of life; in Your presence *is* fullness of joy; at Your right hand *are* pleasures forevermore" (Psalm 16:11 NKJV). Joy is present in God's presence. We rob ourselves of so much when we settle for curling up in despair. Spending time with our Heavenly Father, who loves us and wants to help us, gives us joy. Joy isn't about our circumstances. It's about God's presence in those dark days.

Sweet friend, will you reach out to God's lifeline of hope? Hope isn't about getting our prayers answered favorably. Hope is knowing God is in control, and His mercy and grace will bring us out of the darkness into His marvelous light. Don't allow your feelings or the pain to steal your hope. It is a gift from the Father.

Can you lean into Jesus and allow His light to shine on you today? Pain and illness are hard, but we have the power of God on our side. Let your Heavenly Daddy pick you up today.

Seek the Lord and His strength;
Seek His face evermore!
1 Chronicles 16:11 NKJV

Lord Jesus, I've allowed life to bring me down. Bring me out of this darkness and fill me with hope and joy. Let me always put You before me. In Your name I pray. Amen.

Day 24

The Power of Persistence

Now He was telling them a parable to show that at all times
they ought to pray and not become discouraged.
Luke 18:1 NASB

Exhausted and sore, I lay down on my bed for a short rest. I was surprised how quickly I recuperated after cleaning the bathtub for the first time since surgery. I eagerly made phone calls and posted my achievement on Facebook. I didn't think I could bend over that tub and scrub it with a back full of metal, but God gave me the strength to do it.

I felt a sense of accomplishment each time I entered the bathroom, inhaled the scent of cleanliness, and ran my hand across the smooth shower wall.

I avoided certain activities, like cleaning the bathtub, because I feared additional pain. When you live with pain, both fear and pain become obstacles, preventing you from moving forward with life. We must push past the pain physically and push past the fear mentally. Whether it's cleaning the bathtub, changing the sheets, taking a walk, or going to church, our muscles must move.

Our faith muscles must move also, or we will experience spiritual atrophy. We're not talking about climbing Mount Everest. We must take one step. Take one step in pain, one step in prayer, and one step in faith. Persistent baby steps turn obstacles into stepping stones.

Jesus knew we'd become discouraged, so He gave us a parable about a persistent widow in Luke 18. She continually pleaded with a wicked judge, seeking justice from her adversary. Women had no social standing in that culture. Widows had no one to assist them and no money to bribe the judge. She stood outside his court, probably held in a tent, and cried out for mercy.

This judge didn't fear God or respect people, but he finally gave her justice because she kept bothering him. He was afraid she would give him a bad reputation.

Unlike this widow, we are the King's kids. Jesus is our advocate in heaven, continually interceding for us. We have a special connection through Him, one that doesn't require bribes. He goes before the Father on our behalf out of love.

God is holy, loving, and merciful, the exact opposite of this ungodly judge. How much more will God answer our prayers? "Now, will God not bring about justice for His elect who cry out to Him day and night, and will He delay long for them?" (Luke 18:7 NASB).

We think God delays, but He is already working. He's healing one nerve at a time. He's healing one cell at a time. He's strengthening one muscle at a time. Pray persistently when you don't see God's hand, because He's still working.

Pain is the persistent reminder to pray persistently. Like an alarm clock buzzing, it wakes you up from your sleep. It interferes with your activities, but instead of hitting the snooze button, cry out to God once again.

Prayer exercises our faith muscles, but we must pray believing. We must pray in faith and not in doubt. After telling this parable, Jesus asked if He would find faith on the earth when He returns. Jesus knows it will be hard to walk by faith in these last days.

As we persist in pain, persist in prayer, and persist in faith, we resist the enemy. He wants to discourage us. He doesn't want us to achieve success in activities that used to be so easy, because it gives us the sense of overcoming. It tells us God hasn't forgotten us, and His strength belongs to us.

The enemy creates roadblocks because he doesn't want us to persist in prayer or faith. He fights us each time we bow our heads and determine to believe God has a plan for us.

How does this parable about the persistent widow speak to you? How do you need to persist?

I challenge you to add an additional prayer time to your day. It doesn't need to be long, just enough time to worship Him and persist in making your requests. We can never pray too much. Prayer ushers us into the presence of God. He wants us to enter His throne room with boldness.

> Let us therefore come boldly to the throne of
> grace, that we may obtain mercy and find grace
> to help in time of need.
> Hebrews 4:16 NKJV

Heavenly Father, it's me again, but I know You love hearing from me. I need Your healing touch. I need Your grace and mercy. Thank You. In Jesus' name. Amen.

Day 25

When Joy Fades

Dear brothers and sisters, when troubles of any kind come your way, consider it an opportunity for great joy. For you know that when your faith is tested, your endurance has a chance to grow. So let it grow, for when your endurance is fully developed,you will be perfect and complete, needing nothing.
James 1:2–4 NLT

Have you traversed a season so traumatic that joy fled, leaving nothing but an empty, deserted shell? Perhaps, pain has emptied you of all things joyful as it did to me.

Do you ever wonder why God doesn't show more mercy to your fragile body? I believed God's mercy would bring me through my surgery with minimal pain and no complications. When the reality of the situation set in, my faith wavered. The healing was extremely slow, and even now, I live with reminders of spine surgery.

Disappointment loomed over me like a dark storm cloud. I stayed awake at night with my legs running, and my joy ran away too. Things could have been worse, but I focused on the circumstances and not Christ.

The Holy Spirit produces the fruit of joy within us. The world conflates joy with happiness, but Christians can have joy even in the worst storms.

Look at our focal verse. I selected the *New Living Translation (NLT)* because the wording shows us more clearly what I discovered. James doesn't say the trial counts as joy. Instead, joy comes from the opportunity of the trial.

Seasons of trials come to test our faith. The devil means it for evil, but God uses it for good (Genesis 50:20). As we weather the storms of life, our endurance grows, fulfilling God's purpose for the trial.

Biblical joy is a fruit of the Spirit (Galatians 5:22). It isn't based on our circumstances, but on what Jesus has done on the cross, and what He does in our lives today. Let's examine closely what Jesus calls joy. "Fixing our eyes on Jesus, the pioneer and perfecter of faith. For the joy set before him he endured the cross, scorning its shame, and sat down at the right hand of the throne of God" (Hebrews 12:2 NIV).

His joy came on Resurrection Day, on Sunday. He looked beyond the shame and agony of the cross on Friday, and He looked forward to conquering sin, death, and hell on Sunday.

My friend, Jesus's joy centered around dying for us and saving us. Our salvation brought Jesus joy. How amazing is that?

Joy isn't based on anything earthly, so nothing earthly can steal our joy. We must keep our eyes focused on Jesus, not on pain or anything earthly. As I write that sentence, I realize it's easy to say when I'm not in pain, but it's the truth.

The apostle Peter gives us more insight into changing our perspective. He wrote:

> Dear friends, do not be surprised at the fiery ordeal that has come on you to test you, as though something strange were happening to you. But rejoice inasmuch as you participate in the sufferings of Christ, so that you may be overjoyed when his glory is revealed.
> 1 Peter 4:12–13 NIV

Peter tells us not to be surprised by trials. When life is going on like normal, a trial is an unwelcome surprise.

Peter tells us we're participating in the sufferings of Christ. This is a reason for rejoicing. I often considered the thirty-nine lashes with a cat of nine tails that ripped open the back of Christ. It contained several leather strips with sharp pieces of metal or bone.

The joy set before Jesus throughout all His beatings and crucifixion laid ahead of Him. He focused on Sunday, not on Friday's pain.

When we see Christ in His full glory, we'll be overjoyed. All our suffering will never compare to the glory revealed at that time (Romans 8:18).

Let's keep our joy alive, not allowing pain, fear, stress, or especially the devil to steal it. Let's switch our perspective and our focus. Like Christ, our eyes are on the future. Since His joy came from giving us salvation, our joy should surround our salvation too.

Friend, I leave you with the words of Christ as He spoke to His disciples with His impending death at hand.

I have told you this so that my joy may be in you
and that your joy may be complete.
John 15:11 NIV

Jesus, thank You for giving me Your joy, and help me focus on the spiritual as I learn to endure. In Your name I pray. Amen.

Day 26

Trusting Fully in the Lord

Trust in the Lord with all your heart,
And lean not on your own understanding;
In all your ways acknowledge Him,
And He shall direct your paths.
Proverbs 3:5–6 NKJV

Lying on the exam table, I prayed when the nurse left the sterile room. I sensed they weren't pleased with the mammogram or sonogram.

"Please don't let me need a biopsy, Lord!" I didn't have time for more appointments, treatments, or sickness. I wanted to move forward with life.

I finally felt well enough physically to return to my speaking ministry. I had plans to call churches and inquire about potential speaking events. *I don't need this now.*

God spoke to me, giving me our focal verse. God wants us to be submissive to Him. I want to be in control, but God is our Heavenly Father, and He commands submission.

I trusted God, but doubt lingered in the deep recesses of my heart. The spine surgery left me with a shaky faith. I was no longer the "faith that walks on water" lady. I prayed, "I want to trust You with all my heart, but I need Your help."

If you are not trusting God with all your heart, let that be your prayer also. It's hard because we allow overwhelming doubt, discouragement, and disappointment to smother our trust in God. We fear what He has in mind, because God has the most unusual plans, which aren't always easy.

When we trust in the Lord with all our hearts, we must put our faith into action. Faith isn't a mindset. It's a lifestyle. We must walk out our faith.

Trusting God completely is difficult when our emotions tell us something different. Emotions are real, but they lie. God's Word speaks truth; our feelings don't.

Fear had me going through cancer treatments already, and I wasn't ready for that. Hadn't I been through enough? I needed a break!

"Lean not on your own understanding." That speaks to those feelings and the fearful thoughts fueling them. It speaks to the doubts the enemy plants in our minds. Trust fully in God and not in ourselves.

I got God's message as the nurse returned and left again. I wanted to go home and be done with all of this, but God had other plans. They needed to do a biopsy. God impressed upon me to go through with it. Don't you hate it when God's plans aren't your own? By this time, God had convinced me to have the biopsy. When they told me they would schedule it, I felt disappointed because I wanted to get it over with.

Let's continue unpacking this treasure so we can comprehend this truth. Submission isn't giving up our best life. It's accepting God's best life for us.

"In all your ways, acknowledge Him." In every decision we make, check in with God. My life will run more smoothly when God is in control. He is already in control, but I get in His way with my own ideas, the ones I don't discuss with Him. Checking in with God is liberating. Let our loving Father be in charge because His plans far exceed ours.

Sound the band, because here comes the promise guaranteed to us when we do all the above. When we trust God with all our hearts, and we stop leaning on our own understanding, plus acknowledge Him in all our ways, He will direct our paths. That promise brings me comfort. I don't have to worry about making the wrong decision because I am on His path.

I had the biopsy, and it was negative. Thank God! If I had done things my way, I would have declined the biopsy and lived with a fear in the back of my mind. Now, I don't have to live with that nagging fear haunting me in the middle of the night.

God's paths can include pain and sickness, but His paths don't take us into areas of fear and discouragement. His paths include a future and a hope (Jeremiah 29:11).

> He who trusts in his own heart is a fool,
> But whoever walks wisely will be delivered.
> Proverbs 28:26 NKJV

Lord God, help me depend solely on You with all my heart, not just a portion. When I tend to lean on myself, remind me to acknowledge You in all things. Thank You for Your paths, which are better for me. In Jesus's name. Amen.

Day 27

Hope in the Face of Disappointment

For we were saved in this hope, but hope that is seen is not hope; for why does one still hope for what he sees? But if we hope for what we do not see, we eagerly wait for *it* with perseverance.
Romans 8:24–25 NKJV

Have you ever experienced a trial when God is silent? We often associate His silence with the assumption that He isn't working on our behalf. The burden of those disappointments weighed heavily on me for a long time. My energy level had tanked out on top of everything else. I wanted to pick up my laptop and write again, but I lacked the enthusiasm to follow through with it.

The enemy tried to convince me that my ministry was over. I tried not to believe it, but fatigue kept me from putting any effort into writing, and I didn't see God changing anything.

Friend, He still cares, and He isn't done with you. When God is silent, He isn't still. How do we handle God's silence when we desperately need Him?

Mary and Martha heard only silence as they watched their brother die with no sign of Jesus. When Lazarus, their brother whom Jesus loved, became ill, they immediately sent a messenger to Jesus. They expected Him to come and heal their brother.

When Jesus finally arrived, the sisters didn't hide their disappointment. Martha met Jesus first. "Martha said to Jesus, 'Lord, if You had been here, my brother would not have died'" (John 11:21 NKJV).

In other words, "It's Your fault my brother died, Jesus." Martha firmly believed Jesus would have healed Lazarus. With great boldness, Martha confronted Jesus. Do we confront Jesus with our disappointments? Do we have those conversations in our prayers?

Notice Jesus did not rebuke Martha for her accusation. He already knows how we feel, so why not have an honest conversation with Him? What if we did this at the first hint of disappointment, instead of allowing our disappointment to grow into hopelessness?

When you suffer long, and Jesus is quiet, have you ever found yourself withdrawing from Him? Mary was usually eager to meet Jesus, but she remained in the house until Martha called her to see Him. Mary responded with the same accusatory tone as Martha. Jesus disappointed both sisters with His delay, and they didn't hide their feelings.

Mary still fell at the feet of Jesus, even in the face of grief (John 11:32). This is a posture of worship. Mary still worshiped Jesus after He didn't come in time to heal Lazarus.

If you face great suffering, disappointment, and delays today, don't shut Jesus out. You may not feel like worshipping Him, but once you do, my friend, you'll feel better.

During my recovery, I lost my praise. Yes, I still shouted, "Amen!" and "Hallelujah!" But my praise lacked fervency. One day, I realized that, and I made a point to praise my Lord, and I felt better. Praise consoles the pain.

Mary and Martha grieved. Delay and disappointment confused them. Their faith turned to doubt, but they witnessed the greatest miracle Jesus did on earth.

Jesus asked Martha to roll away the stone from Lazarus's grave. Jesus yelled out for Lazarus to come forth. Lazarus walked out of the tomb.

Can we learn to hold onto hope during the discouragement of great suffering? Look at today's verses. It says hope that is seen isn't hope. We walk by faith and not by sight (1 Corinthians 5:7). Mary and Martha didn't see Jesus, so they lost hope as Lazarus faded away. We don't see relief, and we also lose hope, but hope isn't seen. Otherwise, why would we hope for it?

Our passage continues by saying if we hope for what we don't see, we eagerly wait for it. We tend to give up on it instead of eagerly waiting, and we certainly lack perseverance.

We eagerly wait for Thanksgiving and Christmas, birthdays and anniversaries, vacations, and good news from the doctor. Can we hope for Jesus with that same anticipation?

Resurrect your hope today. You may not see Jesus coming down the road now, but when Jesus seems late, He is always on time.

But as for me, I watch in hope for the Lord,
I wait for God my Savior;
my God will hear me.
Micah 7:7 NIV

Lord God, I go to a place of hopelessness and think the worst. Help me wait on You because I know You hear my cries. In Jesus's name. Amen.

Day 28

Victorious Through Christ

Yet in all these things we are more than
conquerors through Him who loved us.
Romans 8:37 NKJV

Only five days remained until my first speaking event since spine surgery. I sat in the doctor's office, anticipating a prescription for acid reflux. My doctor asked some questions, and before I sat on the exam table, she asked, "Do you have your gall bladder?"

"Yes," I replied.

She sent me straight to the emergency room. After some tests, they concluded my gallbladder had to come out immediately.

"Let's get it done so I can still speak on Saturday." I felt determined, tired of my health ruling my life. But God had a different plan.

The morning after the surgery, the surgeon came by my room and told me I had to keep a drain in for one week, and no showers. Did I mention it was summer? I quickly realized I couldn't stand before a group of women with fluid draining out of me into a little pouch with nothing more than sponging off sweat.

I also discovered that without a gallbladder, I had extraordinarily little warning about going to the bathroom, which made leaving the house almost impossible. My doctor finally prescribed some medication to help with my digestive issues. But I had to cancel yet one more speaking engagement.

God wants us to know we are more than conquerors, but I didn't feel like a conqueror. Can you relate?

Let's look at our verse in reverse. "Through Him who loved us." This refers to Jesus Christ, who loved us so much that He left the glories of heaven to come to earth. He lived with ridicule, suffered, and died on Calvary's hill for us. He died so we can live.

We are more than conquerors because of His death and resurrection. We stand on His finished work in victory.

A conqueror is victorious and wins the battles. Since we are more than conquerors, we are more than victors.

Here's the thing: *in* all these things, we are more than conquerors. We're not conquerors *over* these things. We're not conquerors *of* these things but *in* them.

"These things" refers to suffering. Let's look back at Romans 8:36 (NKJV). "As it is written: 'For Your sake we are killed all day long; we are accounted as sheep for the slaughter.'"

We don't relate to sheep going to the slaughter, but we know suffering. We know pain so intense it makes us scream. We know about illnesses and treatments. We know about the financial worries of medical bills.

We are more than conquerors *in* the suffering, not *over* it. We pray for healing. God wants us to pray, believing He will heal, but in His sovereignty, He doesn't always heal according to our timetable.

God is sovereign, and His plans don't always match our expectations. How are we conquerors if we're not conquerors over our pain and illnesses? We conquer the temptation to give in to despair rather than living victoriously, no matter our physical condition.

Conquerors take captives. We take every discouraging thought captive and quench the enemy's fiery darts of doubt with the shield of faith. When the enemy whispers lies, tell him a Bible verse like Jesus did. Tell the enemy, "It is written."

We can conquer panic, hopelessness, anxiety, discouragement, and disappointment. Jesus gave us His peace. He is our hope, and we have joy because of Jesus, not our health. The enemy steals these blessings from us, but we are more than conquerors, and we must fight to hold onto them.

After all of my suffering, I know what it means to live like a conqueror.

God conquers our trials, but we conquer the enemy's lies. What should you conquer to overcome the enemy today? Which lies do you believe? How do you feel about God's sovereignty?

As you prepare to fight the enemy's schemes, remember this verse from the apostle John.

> You are of God, little children, and have
> overcome them, because He who is in you is
> greater than he who is in the world.
> 1 John 4:4 NKJV

Heavenly Father, help me understand and accept Your sovereignty. Help me live like a conqueror and not fall victim to the enemy's seeds of doubt. In Jesus's name. Amen.

Day 29

Four Keys to Spiritual Endurance

Therefore we also, since we are surrounded by so great a cloud of witnesses, let us lay aside every weight, and the sin which so easily ensnares us, and let us run with endurance the race that is set before us.

Hebrews 12:1 NKJV

I bundled up with a thick sweater, heavy coat, hat, scarf, and gloves to walk with a new guide dog in wind chills of four degrees. I hated retiring Iva and walking with a white cane. I couldn't wait another year for a home training. I jumped at the first chance to fly to New York to meet Yola, my new guide dog.

Even though Iva remained with us, I couldn't stand losing her as a partner. She had started limping due to a tendon problem and needed some time off her feet. This pushed me like nothing else had before. I pushed my body to see if I could attend guide dog school and the strenuous schedule.

We hadn't taken a vacation in almost three years, and preparing to travel lifted my spirits. I just didn't want to end up in immense pain while there.

Physical endurance is important for our bodies, but spiritual endurance is vital for our souls. *Vines Dictionary* defines endurance as "bearing up courageously under suffering." In this verse, we find four keys to build spiritual endurance.

First, we have the witnesses of the Bible. Job suffered patiently. Joseph endured thirteen long years of trials, not knowing where God was taking him. God commanded Abraham to sacrifice his son. The woman with the issue of blood suffered for twelve years and persevered to reach Jesus.

We keep our hope alive by considering the testimonies of these witnesses who have gone before us.

It's also vital to lay aside any extra weight that slows us down. When a runner races, they wear light clothing, so they don't weigh themselves down. The same is true for us spiritually.

Doubt, discouragement, and disappointment burden us with a heavy load. They keep us depressed, confined to our homes, or even in bed. The enemy knows how detrimental this is to a believer. We have to throw off these weights.

We also have to throw off what's wrong in our lives. Sin interferes with answered prayer and blessings. Sin adds to the weight that isn't sinful, and we won't be able to finish our race.

Finally, we run to win. Our bodies might not be able to run in a race, but this spiritual race is more important. We must build up endurance to win. We win when we say no to anxious thoughts and yes to peace. We win when we take doubts captive and meditate on the Word of God. We win when we don't allow the enemy to steal our joy.

Embers of endurance aren't snuffed out in the ashes. They rise up to become beautiful again.

Are you struggling with spiritual endurance? What weight can you remove? Do you need to repent of sin? What is one way you can run to win today?

The Spirit of the Lord God *is* upon Me,
Because the Lord has anointed Me
To preach good tidings to the poor;
He has sent Me to heal the brokenhearted,
To proclaim liberty to the captives,
And the opening of the prison to *those who are* bound;
To proclaim the acceptable year of the Lord,
And the day of vengeance of our God;
To comfort all who mourn,
To console those who mourn in Zion,
To give them beauty for ashes,
The oil of joy for mourning,
The garment of praise for the spirit of heaviness;
That they may be called trees of righteousness,
The planting of the Lord, that He may be glorified.
Isaiah 61:1–3 NKJV

Heavenly Father, examine me and show me the sin and weight I need to lay aside in order to run with endurance the race of faith. In Jesus's name. Amen.

Day 30

Even If

If we are thrown into the blazing furnace, the God we serve is able to deliver us from it, and he will deliver us from Your Majesty's hand. But even if he does not, we want you to know, Your Majesty, that we will not serve your gods or worship the image of gold you have set up.
Daniel 3:17–18 NIV

How often do you ask, "What if?" You may not ask anyone else, but your mind travels through all sorts of incredible scenarios. I allowed my thoughts to run wild with these questions.

What if this is my new life? I experienced complications after my surgery. Some were short-lived, but some continue today.

What if I can't publish or speak again? The enemy taunted me with this constantly. Publishing costs had greatly increased, and due to my health, I had to cancel several speaking events.

What if I can't wear my blue jeans again? My beloved blue jeans hurt my back, and I couldn't wear them for over one year. I had to live in sweatpants except for the summer months. Try wearing a sweater or a flannel shirt with sweatpants. It doesn't match!

Have you asked similar questions? What are your "What ifs?" Instead of asking, "What if?" declare, "Even if."

Shadrach, Meshach, and Abed-Nego didn't ask, "What if?" They made declarations about God's power. When facing a blazing furnace, they did so with commitment, courage, and confidence.

When the Babylonian king commanded everyone to worship his immense gold image, these three young men refused, so he gave them a second chance. If they didn't comply, they would be cast into a fiery furnace. Our focal verses have their reply to the king. They would never bow down to him or his image.

They knew God was able to deliver them from the blazing fire, but they also knew God was sovereign. God is in total control of all things, and we know sometimes God answers in mysterious ways. These three Hebrews could live with that. They were willing to die for it too.

Previously, in Daniel chapter one, these men, along with Daniel, refused to eat the king's food. In a foreign culture, their commitment to God was bold. They continued to prove that same commitment when they refused to worship this gold image.

The three Hebrews also displayed great courage. They didn't allow fear to interfere with their commitment to God.

They took a firm stand in their faith, confident God would deliver them, even if by death.

It's important we stay committed to God during our fiery trials. We accomplish that by lingering in the Word and praying.

We become discouraged during bouts of pain and illness. The enemy uses discouragement to steal our courage, and fear intrudes into our thoughts. Those feelings make our battles more difficult because we make decisions out of fear.

We must hold onto our confidence in God, not confidence in faith, but in our Heavenly Father. Doubts weaken our faith, and we begin trusting the doctors and treatments more than God.

King Nebuchadnezzar became furious with the three Hebrews, ordering his men to throw them into the furnace. He was surprised to see them walking around unharmed with a fourth man in the fire. In shock, the king realized the fourth man was the Son of God.

They removed the Hebrews from the furnace without any burns or hint of smoke on them. With all the confidence they possessed before in God, their faith received a boost. Look how God rewarded their unwavering faith.

Are you feeling discontented, discouraged, or doubtful? When our lives are disrupted by health problems, the enemy steals our joy, our peace, and our hope. That makes our commitment fragile. We wonder if God really cares, since He hasn't answered our prayers. We get weary in the waiting. Instead of courage, we remain discouraged, and doubt chisels away at our faith.

God is able. Nothing is too hard for Him. Let's rest in His sovereignty like the three Hebrews and say, "Even if."

I challenge you to join me in changing our vocabulary. Let's remove the "what if" questions. Let's learn to live with the same commitment, courage, and confidence Shadrach, Meshach, and Abed-Nego had. Let's say, "Even if."

Heavenly Father, I'm tired of living in doubt and discouragement. I know You are able to do anything, but even if You don't meet my expectations, I will trust Your plan. Fill me with commitment, courage, and confidence. In Jesus's name. Amen.

Thank you!

If you have been encouraged by this book, will you please leave a review on Amazon. Your review helps this book reach more readers than you might imagine.

About the Author

Carolyn Dale Newell is a bestselling and award-winning author and dynamic speaker who empowers women to break free from emotional strongholds and embrace lives transformed by faith. With eight published books to her name—including the beloved *Guide Dog Tales* devotional series and *Faith That Walks on Water*, a devotional journal—Carolyn's writing is infused with depth, encouragement, and the wisdom gained from her personal journey.

A passionate student of Scripture, Carolyn delights in exploring the riches of God's Word and sharing its profound truths with her readers. She has earned a certificate in Biblical and Theological Foundations and serves as a contributor for iBelieve.com, inspiring women with her insightful articles.

Carolyn is a proud member of the Advanced Writers and Speakers Association (AWSA) and is certified as an AWSA P.O.W.E.R. speaker, bringing her message of hope and resilience to audiences.

Despite living with blindness and chronic pain, Carolyn encourages women as they navigate their own journeys of hardship, offering comfort and wisdom drawn from her own experiences. She resides in the scenic Blue Ridge Mountains of Virginia with her husband, Tim, and their two loyal Black Labrador retrievers—her current and retired guide dogs.

To learn more about Carolyn Dale Newell and explore her books, speaking events, and resources, visit her online at www.amountainoffaith.com.

You can also find her on Facebook at A Mountain of Faith Women's Ministry and on YouTube at Carolyn Dale Newell Author.

Home - amountainoffaith.com

amountainoffaith.com

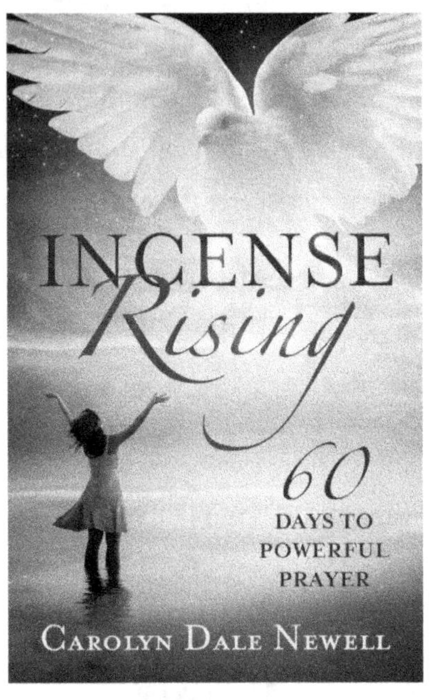

Incense Rising: 60 Days to Powerful Prayer

Deepen your spiritual life through a sixty-day journey into Scripture that explores the riches of prayer. *Incense Rising* helps you identify hindrances to your petitions while teaching you to replace dull routines with fervent, promise-based prayers. By embracing humility and heartfelt worship, you will overcome doubt and draw closer to God in your most important daily conversation.

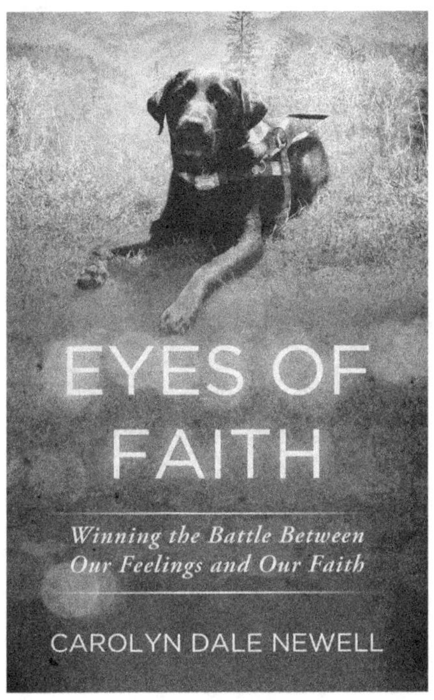

Eyes of Faith: Winning the Battle Between Our Feelings and Our Faith

Eyes of Faith will help you overcome fear, worry, and doubt by discerning truth from deception and embracing God's promises. You will discover how to exchange negative emotions for faith, hope, and peace through Scripture. Cultivate a deeper dependence on God as you learn about your identity as a beloved child of the King.

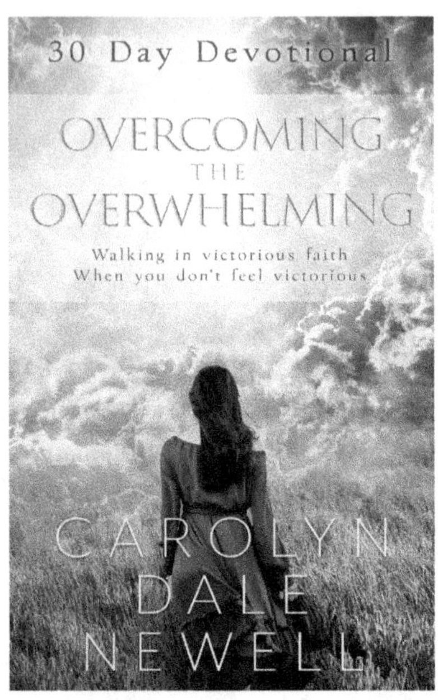

Overcoming the Overwhelming: Walking in Victorious Faith When You Don't Feel Victorious

Overcoming the Overwhelming is a guiding light for those facing life's challenges, offering inspiration to persevere through adversity. Gain insight into spiritual warfare and uncover joy, peace, and strength amid struggles while learning to walk in unwavering faith. This book empowers you to exchange helplessness for hope and experience God's love and acceptance, even in your weakest moments.

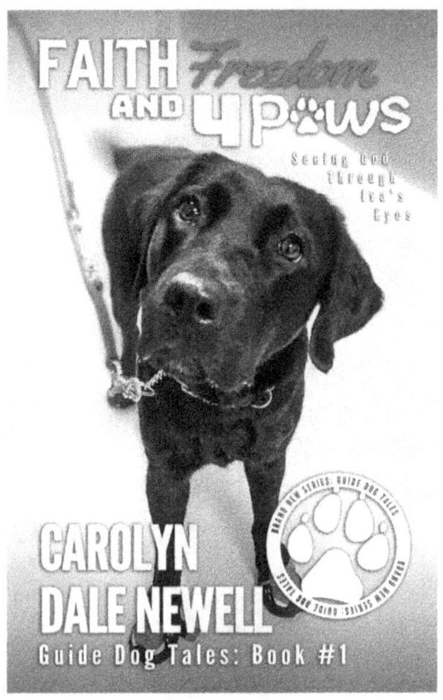

Faith, Freedom, and 4 Paws: Seeing God Through Iva's Eyes
Guide Dog Tales series, book 1

This collection of thirty devotionals follows Carolyn and her guide dog, Iva, offering unique insights into the lives of the visually impaired and the parallels to Christian faith. You will explore the guide dog training process and learn how to deepen your relationship with God, overcome doubt and fear, and pray with confidence. The book's stories inspire readers to walk boldly in faith and find assurance in God's guidance during uncertain times.

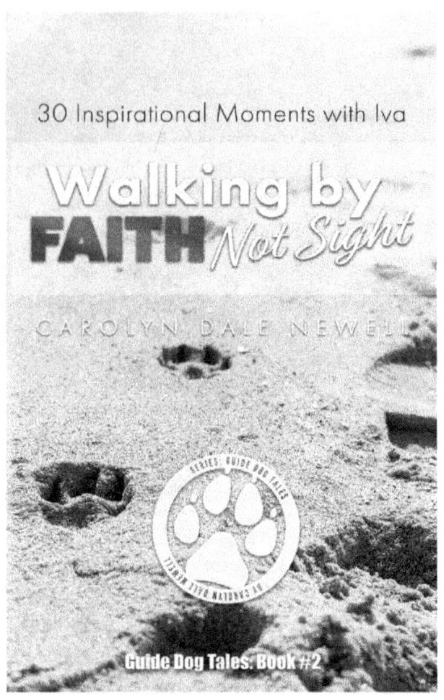

Walking By Faith, Not Sight: 30 Inspirational Moments with Iva

Guide Dog Tales series, book 2

This collection of thirty light-hearted devotionals pairs inspiring stories about Iva with Scripture and prayer prompts to help you find spiritual insight and encouragement. Each devotion is designed to strengthen your faith and guide you through life's challenges with God leading each step. You'll discover practical ways to overcome fear, embrace growth, and approach God with genuine confidence.

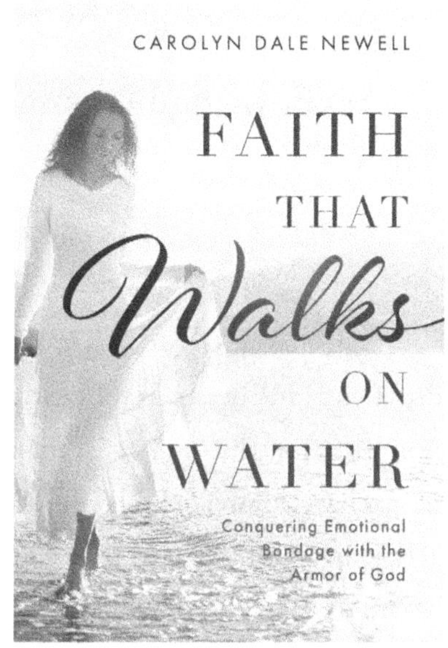

Faith That Walks on Water: Conquering Emotional Bondage with the Armor of God

This sixty-day devotional journal is designed to help you face life's challenges by addressing emotions like fear, worry, and discouragement with practical, scriptural strategies. Through relatable stories and thoughtful prompts, you'll discover how to create your own battle plan to overcome obstacles and deepen your faith. Each devotional guides you to reflect, pray, and take meaningful steps toward experiencing God's love and strength in your daily walk.

Acknowledgments

Thanks to Andrea Lende and her team at Beatitudes Publishing for walking alongside me through this book's publishing process. I could not have completed this project without your support, design, and input. It has truly been a blessing to work with you ladies.

Thanks to the following groups for encouraging me and sharing ideas throughout the writing and marketing process: Book Marketing Pro Academy, Advanced Writers and Speakers Association, and Speak Up Growth Groups.

Thanks to Jennifer Bryant for keeping my website functioning and for her beautiful designs that help this message reach the world.

www.ingramcontent.com/pod-product-compliance
Lightning Source LLC
LaVergne TN
LVHW010947110826
845149LV00015B/3248

* 9 7 8 1 9 6 2 5 8 1 8 4 4 *